the OPHTHALMOLOGIST
and OCULARIST
explore the

Techniques of ANOPHTHALMIC COSMESIS

Techniques of ANOPHTHALMIC COSMESIS

Selected papers and discussion from the Seventeenth Annual Meeting of the American Society of Ocularists, Dallas, Texas.

Edited by
Pierre Guibor, M.D.
Marsha Guibor, C.O.

Published by
Symposia Specialists
MEDICAL BOOKS

STRATTON INTERCONTINENTAL MEDICAL BOOK CORPORATION
381 Park Avenue South, New York, New York 10016

Library of Congress Catalog
Card No. 75-8433

ISBN 0-88372-029-9

Symposia Specialists
MIAMI, FLORIDA 33161

Printed in the U.S.A.

Contents

Orbital Tumors

Congenital Deformities

III. Facial and Systemic

Tumors

Trauma

Aging

I. Lids

- Upper Lids
- Lower Lids

Reduction of Upper Eyelid Ptosis with the Prosthesis, with Special Attention to a recently Devised, More Effective Method

Lee Allen

The problem of ptosis over artificial eyes has probably existed from the first time the rectus muscles were imbricated over a large, truly spherical implant in Tenon's capsule. In a 1937 paper Paul Gougelman [1] stated, "Besides, a large implant invariably destroys the fold of the upper lid and produces apparent ptosis." As early as 1929, Pierre Gougelmann [2] made the following observation:

> Instead of being pleased as I had expected, she objected to a slight difference between the upper lid of the artificial eye as compared to that of the natural eye. Close examination showed that she was entitled to her criticism, but to be able to produce the effect she desired was beyond the power of any mortal.
>
> I have mentioned this case because it is typical of many. The upper lid of the artificial eye often appears to hand over the eye in contrast to the fold of the lid in the natural eye giving the appearance of a slight drooping of the lid. I have repeatedly attempted to overcome this difficulty by adapting a fuller eye, but the fullness thus produced is unnatural and far less pleasing than the original condition. Whether this condition is due to a slight paralysis of the muscle, I do not know. If it is possible to overcome this condition, it would be a welcome relief for such oversensitive patients.

Apparently, many surgeons and ocularists still believe that marked ptosis over artificial eyes cannot be reduced adequately by prostheses. As recently as 1970, Beard, in a chapter on blepharoptosis [3], stated,

---

Lee Allen, Department of Ophthalmology, College of Medicine, University of Iowa Hospitals and Clinics, Iowa City.

"Attempts at elevating the lid by the fitting of a large prosthesis will give disappointing results." Beard probably would have mentioned that the eyelid can be elevated by modifying the shape rather than the size of the prosthesis – without disappointing results – if he had been fully informed about the modern, complex method that will be described later.

I have been writing and lecturing for 21 years on this subject as one of several very effective and important new principles for reducing or correcting cosmetic defects by modifying the forms of the prostheses. Unfortunately for most of the patients like the one reported by Pierre Gougelmann – and the many with truly disfiguring ptosis, it seems that very few ocularists have bothered to learn the method. Patients once had no choice but to live with the ptosis or have surgery. Now, I believe more than 95% of the obvious ptoses can be corrected to a very acceptable point by shaping the prostheses.

Several years ago, Robert Scott was especially impressed by an example I presented in a short motion picture. He tried the method on his own ptosis patients and, having found that it works, has become an advocate. We may hope that all certified ocularists will learn to apply these principles correctly so that ptosis over prostheses will almost become a thing of the past.

Promulgation of the knowledge of the complex principles for correcting ptosis will depend upon aroused interest on everyone's part, effective motivation, advanced training of ocularists and complete cooperation between ophthalmologists and ocularists.

It may not be essential to know the causes and characteristics of various kinds of ptosis in order to reduce them with prostheses since all are reduced by applying the same basic fitting principles, but an informed ocularist may be better prepared to handle his cases and to contribute to further advances in the future. It is helpful to be aware of the differences between persistent, temporary and progressive ptosis and to anticipate that some patients will require early and rather frequent refitting while others will not likely need refitting except for age changes. This knowledge will also help greatly in the ocularists' rapport with ophthalmic surgeons.

Classification of Types of Ptosis

Pseudoptosis

From the ocularists' standpoint, pseudoptosis occurs over poorly fitted prostheses, over microphthalmos, endophthalmos and phthisical globes. When it is of simple form and of minimal extent, it will disappear merely upon fitting with a traditional artificial eye.

There are several types of true ptosis which may be categorized in relation to duration and character.

Persistent Ptosis

Ptoses from accidental or surgical trauma, some neurological and some congenital causes will persist and continue to require special prostheses for full correction. Eventually all may be expected to require refitting due to changes which typically appear with advancing age.

Temporary Ptosis

The largest amount of healing takes place in about four or five weeks after eye removal surgery. Some ptoses will persist for many months but will recede with time. We may classify these as "temporary." They might be caused by edematous tissues in the orbit pressing forward against the upper edge of the tarsus to roll the margin of the upper eyelid forward and downward. As the edema subsides and the tissue mass reduces, the tissues just behind the tarsus drop backward, making room for the upper eyelid to roll back and upward. The ptosis can then be reduced to an acceptable level in many cases with properly designed prostheses. These cases may be even better corrected after further healing.

Patients who have deep hemorrhage or presumed deep hemorrhage in the orbit show exactly the same effect as edema, and the course of regression can be as long or longer.

Some rare patients with edema or hemorrhage require, in the beginning, a shelf (to be detailed later) to support the upper eyelid. The shelf can be removed after one or two years in some of these cases. The impression might be that the shelf corrected the basic problem, but I believe the shelf only helps direct the healing in favorable ways. Caution should be exercised regarding doing any kind of irreversible ptosis surgery in such cases because of the probability of having spontaneous disappearance of the ptosis. If surgery is done, there might be overcorrection of the ptosis.

Temporary ptosis may also be drug-induced, as in steroid myopathy, or it can be caused by inflammation or infection.

Custom-fitted conformers may be made for such sockets or cosmetic prostheses can be made and then refitted at intervals until the ptosis is gone.

Intermittent Ptosis

In order for ocularists to avoid frequent refittings or the making of new prostheses, they should know that some ptoses are intermittent. Nothing can be done to the plastic eye to prevent it. After two or more refittings, during which the prosthesis is perhaps made smaller, then larger, then smaller again, there should be consultation with the ophthalmologist regarding the possibility of intermittent ptosis. It should be recognized that it is not the ocularist's fault in such cases when the level of the upper lid changes back and forth within hours or days. Some of the causes are myasthenia gravis, transient Horner's syndrome (with cluster headaches) and paralysis.

Progressive Ptosis and Pseudoptosis

Some ptoses are progressive beyond the typical changes which occur with long wearing of the prostheses. Not all, but many patients will have rather rapid atrophy of the posterior orbital tissues soon after surgery. If such patients are fitted within a few days after eye removal, the prostheses may later tilt backward. The upper lid will drop into a position of pseudoptosis because of reduced support. Proper refitting can correct this.

Regressing edema can give the same kind of changes for similar reasons.

While familial ptosis is usually bilateral, the ptosis over the prosthesis may progress faster than on the unoperated side and need occasional refitting. Unilateral familial ptosis can occur, also requiring repeated refittings.

Neoplasm (lymphoma) can press the eyelid downward progressively and, if recognized, naturally should be treated by the ophthalmologist rather than refitted with larger prostheses. (This is one of many good reasons why the ocularist and ophthalmologist should work cooperatively. It would be best if every prosthesis patient could be seen by the ophthalmologist whenever there are changes which seem to indicate the prosthesis needs refitting.)

The Methods of Ptosis Reduction

The "Larger Prosthesis" Method

In the simplest method, the "corneal" portion of the artificial eye is thrust forward to wedge the eyelids apart (Fig. 1). At the same time the prosthesis is shaped to keep the "iris-cornea-pupillary" segment properly aligned. (The prostheses thus fitted are of the type referred to by Pierre Gougelmann as the "fuller eye" and by Dr. Beard as the "large prosthesis.")

The "larger prosthesis" method can correct pseudoptosis *but not any true ptosis without having the prosthesis become objectionably prominent* (Fig. 2). I have never seen any marked true ptosis even moderately reduced

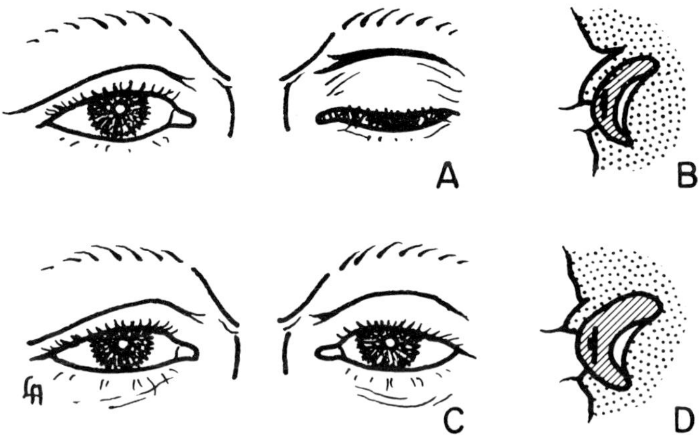

FIG. 1. Reduction of "pseudoptosis" with larger prosthesis. (A) Front-view drawing of typical drooping upper eyelid (OS) over small artificial eye. (B) Cross section showing relationship between prosthesis and tissues. (C) Improved appearance after refitting with larger prosthesis. (D) Cross section showing upper eyelid lifted by forward thrust and resultant wedging effect of artificial eye with larger antero-posterior dimension.

by this means without the prosthesis "looking" downward and greatly depressing the lower eyelid. There is usually discomfort or, at best, a continual sensation of fullness for the wearer.

The Recently Devised, Complex Method

In 1953 a brief description was given of a successful method of reducing ptosis [4] that had been devised at the University of Iowa only a few years earlier. The concept was in a formative stage and has since been perfected and reported. [5-7] It is now being taught in the educational

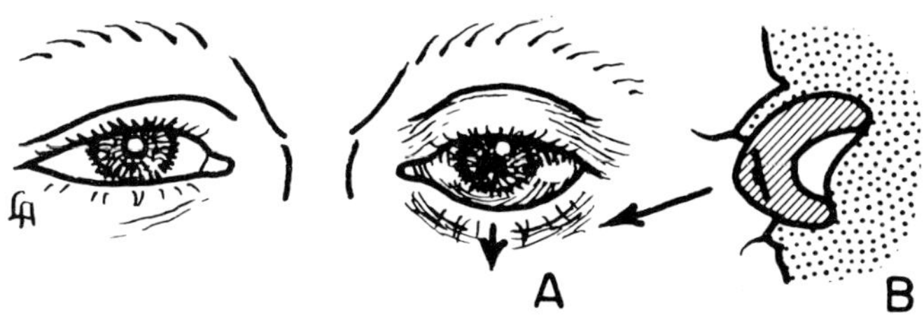

FIG. 2. Typical failure of attempt to correct true ptosis with larger prosthesis. (A) Front-view drawing of upper eyelid ptosis (OS) persisting after refitting of socket with very large artificial eye (note typical objectionable protrusion with undesirable downward gaze). (B) Cross section showing relationship of prosthesis to tissues.

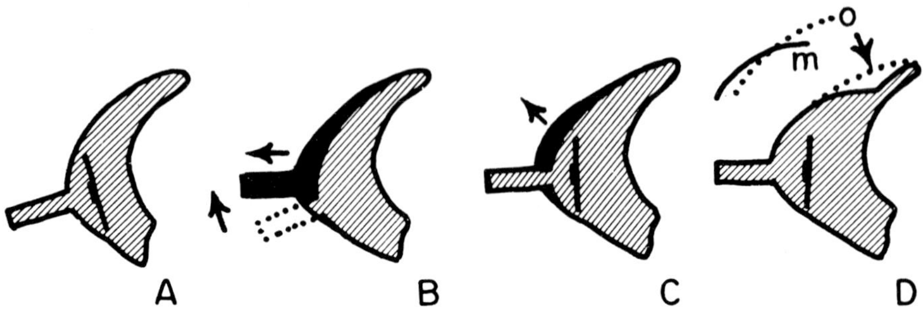

FIG. 3. Cross section drawings of an initial wax pattern (based upon an impression of an eye socket with which ptosis of the upper eyelid is present) and three (of a possible four) successive form modifications of the same pattern toward ptosis reduction. (A) Initial wax pattern which does not reduce any of the ptosis and points downward. (B) Same pattern with "iris-cornea" piece repositioned to gaze straight ahead, "corneal" surface moved forward and blended to upper edge of model, as step 1 of ptosis reduction. (C) Same pattern with added thickness of wax over upper half of "cornea" and upper "limbus," blended onto upper surface of model, as step 2 of ptosis reduction. (D) Wax removed from upper surface (dotted line at 0) to make space into which upper edge of superior tarsus can withdraw, as step 3 of ptosis reduction.

courses of the American Society of Ocularists leading toward certification of its members. I present it as the superior method, one that should become the prosthetic method of choice in the future. To apply this method in the *best* manner, a wax pattern must be made so that it can be freely and quickly altered in size, form and alignment (Fig. 3A). It should be emphasized that it is not absolutely essential for the wax pattern to be based upon an impression of the eye socket, but the modified impression method does give a better physiological filling and thus makes the final prosthesis more comfortable.

Step 1. The anterior surface of the prosthesis ("cornea" and adjacent surface) is extended forward to the same prominence as the cornea of the companion eye (Fig. 3B); thus there is some effect of wedging the eyelid margins apart. The "cornea" is kept at the correct height, pointed correctly and spaced well laterally. This first step, alone, will often correct pseudoptosis. If there is still ptosis, both of the next two steps must be applied.

Step 2. Some excess material is added over the upper half of the "cornea" and across the superior "limbus" only, blending the resulting new surface onto the "sclera" (Fig. 3C). (If this material is added too high, over the "limbus" only, the upper eyelid can actually be "hooked" downward over it – maintaining the appearance of ptosis.)

Step 3. Material is removed from the top surface near the rear edge of the prosthesis to make room for the upper edge of the tarsal plate to swing backward. No material is removed from the upper "limbus," and the resulting new "scleral" surface is blended imperceptibly with the extended "corneal" surface (Fig. 3D). The new plane must be long enough to accommodate the entire vertical width of the tarsus, measuring backward from the level at which the upper eyelid margin should cross the "cornea." This has consistently been 11.5 mm in hundreds of patients in whom we have taken measurements.

The combined effect of steps 1, 2 and 3 is to rotate the upper eyelid upward and backward around its effective "hinges," the insertions of the palpebral ligaments into the bony orbit (Fig. 4A and B). To better understand the principle, the leather-like tarsus, palpebral ligaments and insertions can be compared to an inverted hammock. As in the case of a hammock, if pressure is applied on one edge it rotates away from the

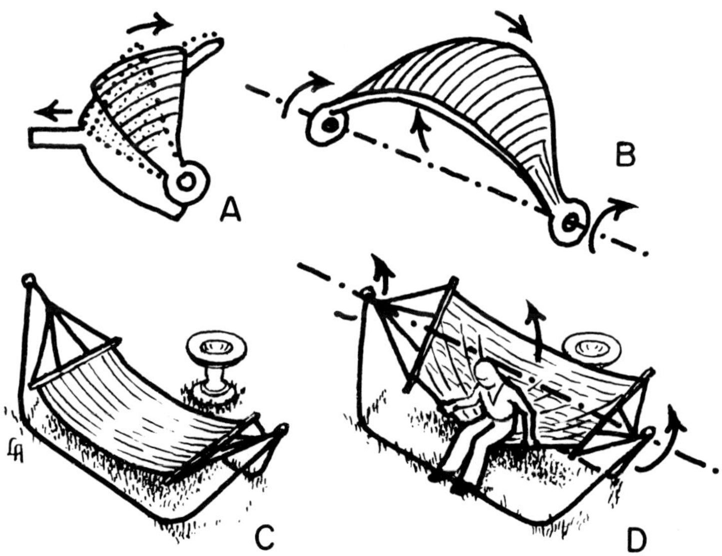

FIG. 4. Schematic drawings of principle of rotation of superior tarsus upward and backward around its "axis" of the points of insertion of the palpebral ligaments into the bony orbit. (A) Side view of ptotic position of upper tarsus (dotted lines) and elevated position (solid lines) after application of steps 1-3 as shown in Figure 3. (B) Perspective view of superior tarsus and palpebral ligaments in elevated position. (C) Hammock to which the superior tarsus may be compared (as an inverted form). (D) Rotation of hammock upon application of force at one side, to be compared to similar rotation of superior tarsus upon upward wedging of eyelid margin.

pressure and around the axis between the points of suspension (Fig. 4C and D). The free edge of the hammock swings out and upward unless something holds it down. In the case of the upper lid, the wedging effect of the extended "cornea" is like the pressure on one side of the hammock (inverted) and the superior "scleral" surface is the force that holds it back. The space made, then, on the top rear surface of the prosthesis (step 3) is like the space into which the free edge of the hammock must swing. If there is still ptosis after the above principles are applied, a fourth step should be carried out.

Step 4. A ridge of material is extended upward from the top rear edge of the prosthesis (Fig. 5A) to have two effects. It must absolutely be kept behind the upper edge of the *newly positioned* tarsus (11.5 mm back from the desired level of the eyelid margin on the "cornea," as stated before). It

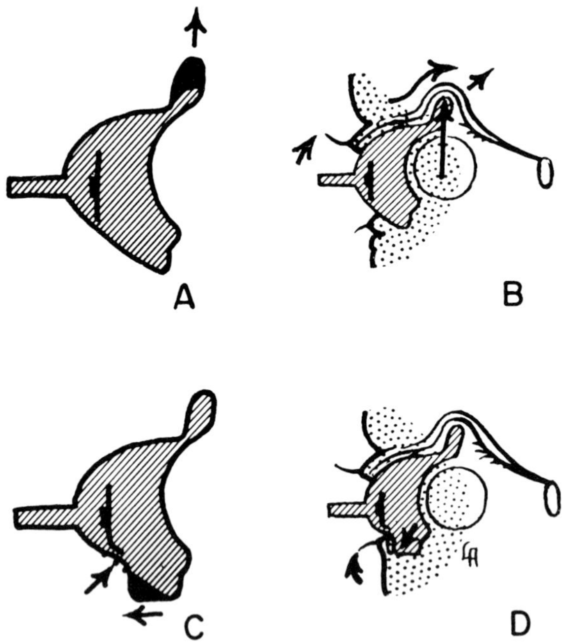

FIG. 5. Cross section drawings of same wax pattern as shown in Figure 3. (A) Material added upward from superoposterior edge to pass beyond upper edge of superior tarsus, as step 4 of ptosis reduction. (B) Mode of action of added material in lifting upper eyelid margin, by buckling levator-Müller's muscle-tarsus continuum and "using up" conjunctiva in superior fornix. (C) Changes in shape of inferoanterior edge of wax pattern to reduce sag of center of lower eyelid. (D) Mode of action of changes in rotating inferior tarsus upward to overcome sagging.

must extend into the superior fornix in order, first, to use up any excess conjunctiva and, second, to make a bend in Müller's muscle and the levator, thus effectively shortening the span of the tarsus-Müller's muscle-levator continuum. Taken together, these two effects help to further lift the upper eyelid margin (Fig. 5B).

The height and thickness of the added ridge will vary with both the available or potential space above the upper fornix and the amount of material needed for the desired effect. In some sockets, there is not enough space to allow any ridge at all. If one is added, the effect is that the prosthesis pushes itself downward unfavorably. It must then be removed.

In other sockets, ridges commonly 4 mm high and 3 mm thick can be used. In rare cases, even higher and thicker ridges can be used. The size limit comes at the point beyond which any more mass will push the prosthesis downward and out of its proper position against the posterior wall of the socket. When this point has been reached, material must be removed from the ridge being added until the prosthesis is no longer displaced.

Step 5. When the first four steps have been completed and the ptosis is reduced to an acceptable level, deformities of the contours of either or both of the eyelid margins may be noted. As one common example, the lower eyelid is likely to sag badly. Nearly always, this can be reduced until it is not noticed by correctly applying the appropriate mechanical principles for elevating a lower lid margin with the prosthesis, as described in earlier publications [5-7] and as illustrated in Figure 5C and D. The fitting of the prosthesis is not complete until these other defects are also corrected or effectively reduced.

Step 6. The final touches can be given by reducing some remaining defects with cosmetic optics in spectacle lenses, as also described elsewhere [5-7].

Demonstration of Correction by the Complex Method in a Patient. An example of full correction of a severe ptosis is shown in Figures 6-13. A 43-year-old woman had an enucleation, OS, with primary placement of the new, larger, quasi-integrated, muscle cone Iowa implant [8-10]. Marked ptosis is rarely seen with this implant, but two months after surgery, she returned (for custom fitting of the cosmetic prosthesis) with an extreme ptosis of the upper eyelid, OS, and poor tonus of the lower eyelid.

Snellen reform shapes (as represented by stock artificial eyes) are never fitted in our department. Only custom prostheses prepared by the modified impression method are fitted to all eye sockets, regardless of what types of eye removal surgery – with or without implant – are

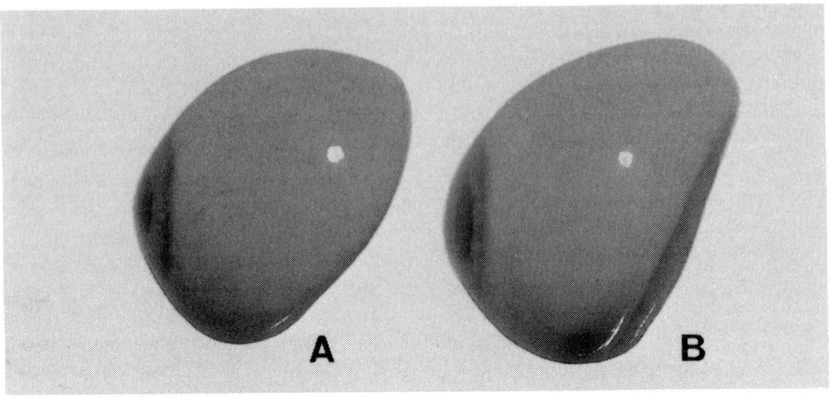

FIG. 6. Traditional plastic artificial eyes. (A) Moderate size, first tried in patient shown in Figure 7A. (B) "Larger prosthesis," next tried in same patient, as shown in Figure 7B.

presented. However, in this case, for didactic purposes only, we placed the plastic eye (Fig. 6A) in the socket to demonstrate the marked ptosis which would be present after the traditional type of eye fitting. The extreme ptosis is shown in Figure 7A. The effect of simply using a "larger prosthesis" (Fig. 6B) is shown in Figure 7B. Besides persistence of the ptosis and drooping lower eyelid, there was an objectionable proptosis.

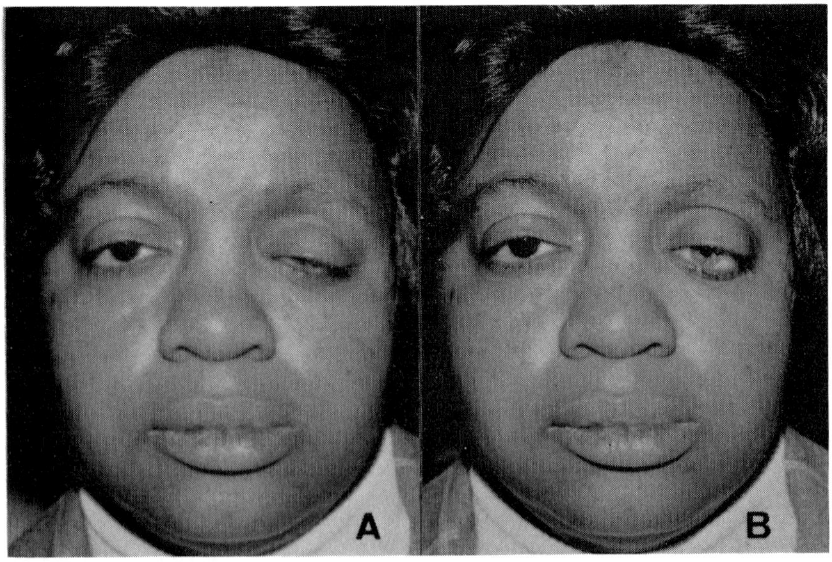

FIG. 7. (A) Patient with marked ptosis wearing traditional prosthesis, OS. (B) Same patient wearing traditional "larger prosthesis."

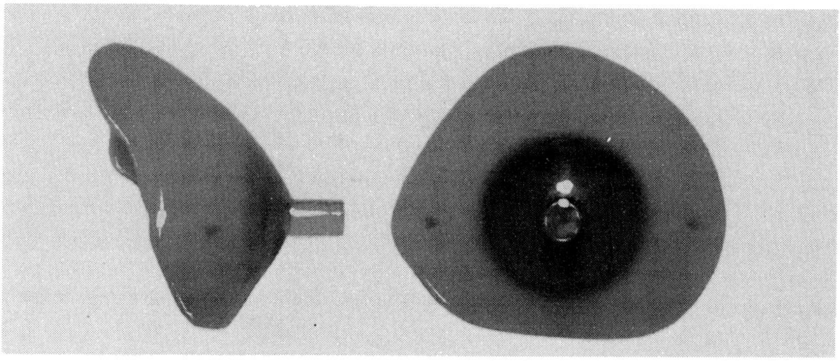

FIG. 8. Unmodified wax pattern for prosthesis based upon impression of eye socket of patient shown in Figure 9.

Following the foregoing demonstrations, the socket was fitted by one of the trainees* in our ophthalmic prosthetics training program, using all of the systematic principles for reduction of ptosis embodied in our special modified impression method of artificial eye fitting.

The first, *unmodified* wax pattern (Fig. 8) did not correct any ptosis, as shown in Figure 9. The fully modified wax pattern (Fig. 10) fully corrected the upper eyelid ptosis and left only a minimal sag in the temporal side of the lower eyelid, as shown in Figure 11.

At this point, the shape of the wax pattern was duplicated exactly in plastic by a molding technique. The plastic eye was colored to match the patient's OD, reprocessed, smoothed and polished. The prosthesis was

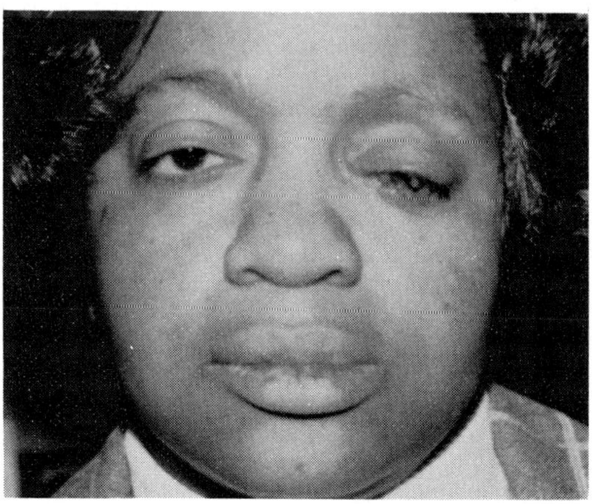

FIG. 9. Same patient as in Figure 7, but wearing unmodified wax pattern shown in Figure 8.

*Mr. Monté Anderson.

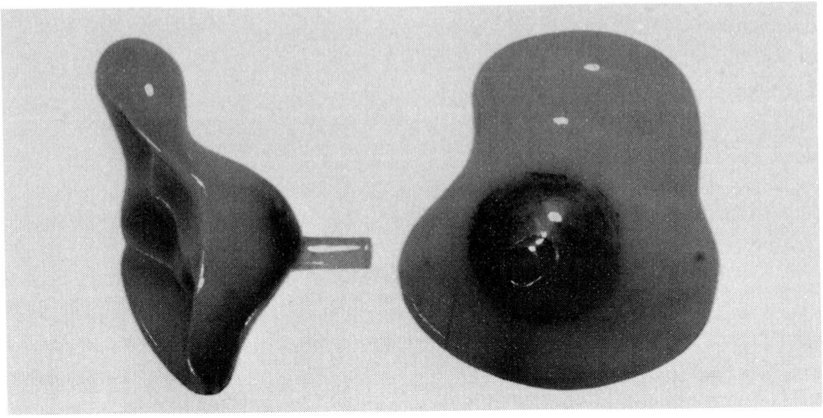

FIG. 10. Fully modified wax pattern (from that shown in Figure 8) for reducing upper eyelid ptosis and other tissue distortions.

placed in the eye socket and the patient was allowed to wear it for approximately a half hour, after which minor adjustments were made by removing small amounts of plastic in critical places and repolishing the entire eye. The final prosthesis (Fig. 12) created a highly satisfactory cosmetic effect, as shown in Figure 13. Besides correcting the upper eyelid ptosis, the prominence was normal, the supraorbital fold gave a normal appearance and the lower eyelid did not sag noticeably. The eyelids, OS, closed upon blinking and it was judged that they would close over the prosthesis during sleep. In spite of the ptosis problems, the motility of the

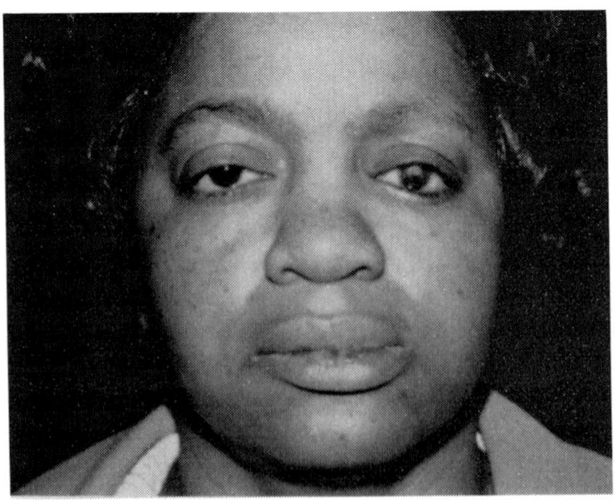

FIG. 11. Same patient as in Figures 7 and 9, but wearing fully modified wax pattern shown in Figure 10.

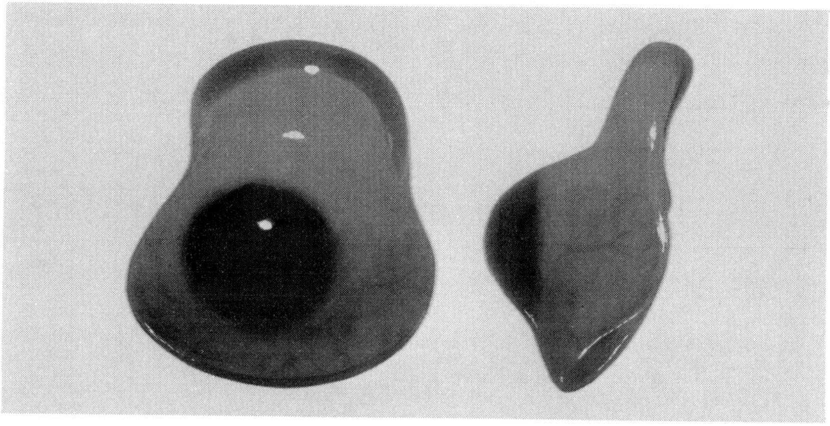

FIG. 12. Finished plastic eye after minor adjustments to improve cosmesis of patient's OS.

prosthesis was good. It was not necessary to use cosmetic optics in this case.

While all pseudoptosis and most ptosis cases can be reduced to the point where they are not recognized or are completely corrected by the complex method, a few true ptoses cannot. Before referring these patients to the ophthalmic surgeons, one or more of the following extreme methods of prosthetic correction might best be tried.

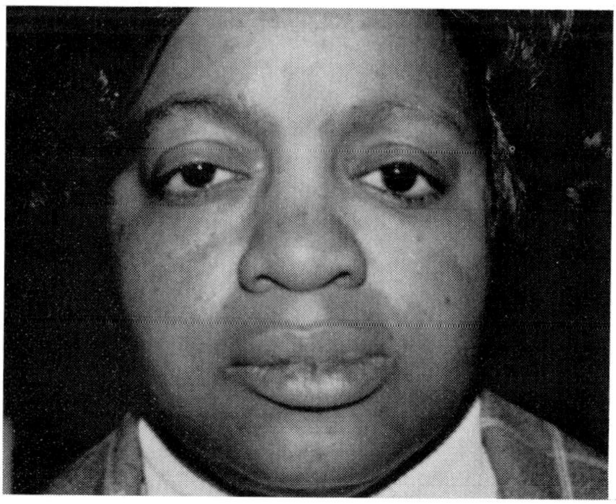

FIG. 13. Same patient as in Figures 7, 9 and 11, but wearing final prosthesis shown in Figure 12.

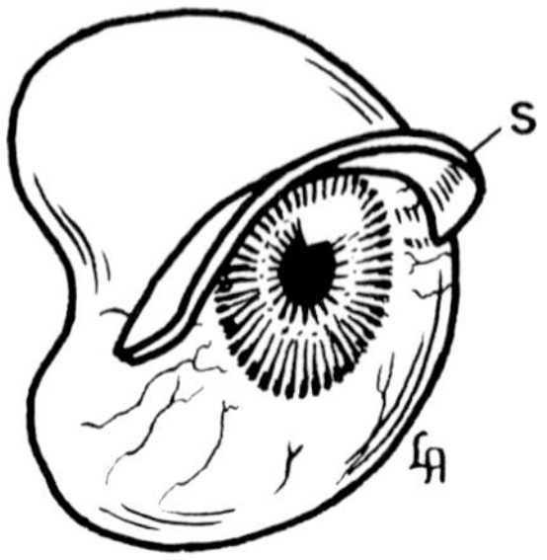

FIG. 14. Drawing of plastic artificial eye, OD, with thin extended shelf to support ptotic upper eyelid.

Extended Shelf

When either the traditional method or the newer, complex method fails to correct ptosis, a thin, transparent shelf [11,12] can be constructed across the front surface of the eye (Fig. 14) to hold the upper eyelid at the desired open position. The shelf can be so thin that it is invisible. This is almost always effective enough to create a very fine illusion of a normal, living eye. The weight of the upper eyelid and the action of the orbicularis muscle often tend to press the eye downward. This can frequently, but not always, be counteracted by adding material at the bottom rear edge of the prosthesis to roll it back upward. If the entire structure is based upon an impression of the eye socket, it can be very comfortable. Even the inhibition of blinking is soon forgotten by the wearer.

The major drawback to the shelf is that the eyelid cannot blink or close. However, it is amazing how few persons will look critically at such a prosthesis if it is well aligned and if it is colored carefully to look like living tissue! Ultimately, however, the shelf is not nearly the equal of the complex method and should not be used if the complex method can be applied.

Incised Shelf

The incised shelf [13] functions in exactly the same manner as the extended shelf, but is used where the upper eyelid is so tight that the plastic eye would otherwise "gaze" upward objectionably. The incised plane can be recessed almost 2 mm without becoming noticeable (Fig. 15).

In some cases, after the prosthesis has been worn for some time, the upper lid becomes more flexible and effectively longer horizontally. If, in addition, there is increased space in the socket, the prosthesis may tilt backward and the upper eyelid may slide forward over the edge of the shelf. Then it is necessary to refit the prosthesis to keep the eyelid on the shelf. However, if other changes in the tissues are favorable, the prosthesis

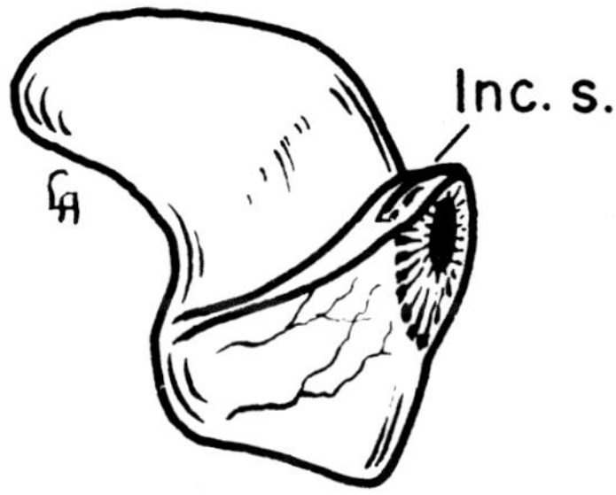

FIG. 15. Drawing of plastic artificial eye, OD, with upper portion incised to leave a shelf for support of a taut upper eyelid with ptosis.

may be refitted without a shelf, as metioned earlier, and the upper eyelid may take a relatively normal position from then on.

Crutch on Spectacle Frame

Some types of ptosis, in occasional patients, can be overcome by a wire or wire spring [14] mounted on spectacle frames (Fig. 16) and extending across into the supraorbital fold to press eyelid tissue upward and backward under the superior rim of the orbit. The device lifts the eyelid and allows blinking in some cases. For some patients it is an effective substitute for surgery.

The crutch has some undesirable features. It is not always possible to hide the wire to the patient's satisfaction. Also, the skin of the eyelid slips downward past the crutch for some, making it necessary occasionally for the patient to adjust the position of contact between the spring and the skin.

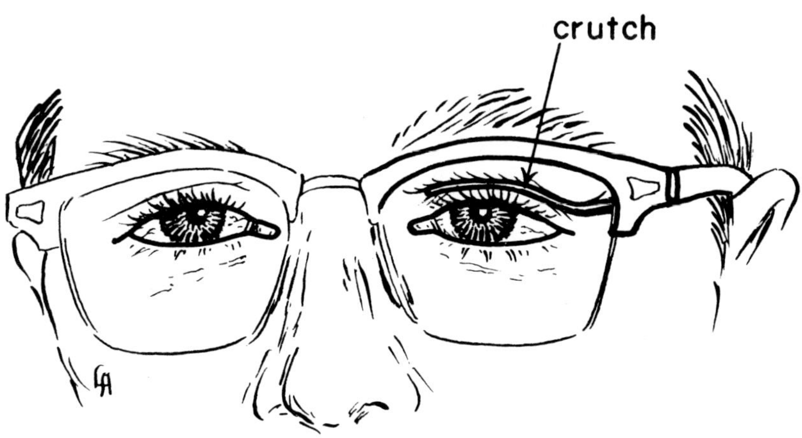

FIG. 16. Drawing of ptosis crutch attached to left side of spectacle frame, to press into supraorbital fold and support upper eyelid, OS.

An Erroneous "Brute Force" Method

I have heard described a method that I find ineffectual and objectionable for attempting to correct ptosis of the upper eyelid. Also, several prosthesis patients have been referred to me who came wearing such prostheses. Material had been built almost straight upward to an extreme height from the superior "limbal" region of the prosthesis (Fig. 17), with the intention of pushing the entire eyelid upward. If the eye fitters involved had known the detailed anatomy of the orbit and what we now know about appropriate mechanical principles, they would have realized that their methods would have the opposite of the desired effect. The mass applied upward pressed forward against the upper edge of the superior tarsus. Because the movement of the upper eyelid is "hinged" around the insertions of the palpebral ligaments in the bony orbit, and because the tarsus has a leather-like firmness, the pressure against the upper edge of the tarsus and the eyelid rotated the eyelid margin forward and downward (Fig. 17C and D). Again, the analogy can be drawn with the inverted hammock, but here the pressure is from the wrong side. Of the several cases that I have seen fitted in this way, none of the ptosis was reduced. The most notable remaining features in every case were the ptosis and an abnormal bulging forward of the tissues between the upper eyelid and the eyebrow. It seems possible there could be stretching of Müller's muscle that could do permanent damage, eventually increasing rather than decreasing the ptosis.

Patients fitted by the "brute force" method are never comfortable. They report great relief when refitted by the complex method. The erroneous "brute force" method *should never be used.*

Surgery

When the complex method has been applied and has failed, it is easy enough to add a shelf or install a wire crutch on spectacle frames to support the eyelid, as already described. According to our experience, a few of those patients with shelves or crutches will continue wearing them indefinitely; some of the others will prefer to have surgical correction. The results have been only moderately good on the latter, probably for the same reasons that the shelves had been needed in the first place.

In contrast to those of our patients who had surgery, two had unexpected and unexplained favorable changes (possibly absorption of hemorrhages) take place which made it possible to remove the shelves after two or more years. After that, only the complex mechanical correction principles in the prosthesis were needed to overcome the slight residual portion of ptosis.

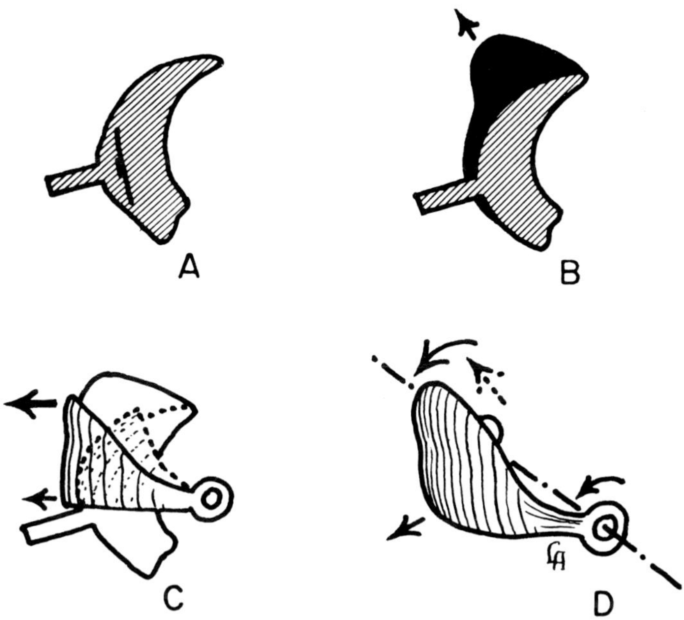

FIG. 17. Schematic drawings showing *erroneous* "brute force" method of attempting to correct upper eyelid ptosis. (A) Cross section of initial wax pattern made from impression of eye socket. (B) Large quantity of wax added (represented in solid black) straight upward from superior "limbus." (C) Side view of superior tarsus and palpebral ligament pushed forward *and held downward* from original position, shown in dotted lines. (D) Perspective view of tarsus and ligaments being rotated by the erroneous method in the wrong direction.

Discussion

It should be emphasized that all but the most rare and difficult cases can be made to look acceptably symmetrical between the sides of the face by using the complex fitting method. That is, they can be made as symmetrical as the average person who may have one eye lower than the other, or more expanse of upper eyelid showing on one side than on the other, without calling attention to the fact. Unfortunately, it will not be possible to have all ptosis patients everywhere fitted this well until all ocularists learn to apply the complex method. This takes special knowledge and months of training, followed by added months of supervised practice. We demand that our trainees remain with us for two years in order to learn all details of form modification, etc. All ocularists must have or develop the skill, the patience and, especially, the persistence to make the best correction possible for every patient.

Frequency of Ptosis over Prostheses

Ptosis can occur in any prosthetic situation from phthisical living globes to eyesockets after complete eye removal. However, severe ptosis has been seen in our clinic more commonly with one specific type of enucleation with spherical implant than with any other eye removal surgery. A systematic listing of the basic types of surgery follows:

1. *Scarred, full-size globes* which require flush-fitting cosmetic shell eyes are no more likely to have associated ptosis than nonscarred eyes.

2. Pseudoptosis is seen with *phthisical globes* more often than true ptosis, although the latter can occur in mild form from the continuing pull of the superior rectus muscle sheath upon the sheath of the levator muscle due to shrinkage of the globe.

3. *Simple enucleation* is more likely to present pseudoptosis than true ptosis. Because of the typical deepening of the supraorbital fold from atrophy of fat and the resulting sucking backward and rotating downward of orbital tissues, a greater expanse of the eyelid is seen both before and after prosthesis fitting than on the companion eye, even though the upper lid margins are at the same level. This expanse makes the eye look a little bit "sleepy." In this type of eye socket, it usually is not possible to completely correct the deep supraorbital fold with prostheses without introducing or exaggerating some other fault, such as limitation of closure of the upper eyelid. Overcorrecting the apparent ptosis very slightly helps because it shortens the expanse of the eyelid seen. But when this is done, a slightly wider open palpebral fissure will often result which must be accepted or rejected by the patient and ocularist. If it is accepted, the "cornea-iris" section may be made slightly large to create a good illusion of space filling.

Sometimes in this simple enucleation (and in any other type of complete eye removal) where the optic nerve has been sectioned with scissors, a ptosis appears that is either impossible or almost impossible to correct with the prosthesis. These are not of the type which results from massive orbital hemorrhage and they do not correct themselves in time. A possible cause is that the superior rectus and the levator muscles have been severely traumatized as a result of surgery.

4. *Enucleation with spherical implant, muscles not imbricated,* has relatively few ptosis results. Forward position of the sphere can be a fitting problem unless some surgical procedure such as that described by Costen [12] is used.

5. *Enucleation with 16- to 18-mm spherical implant, muscles imbricated,* has invariably been accompanied by ptosis, in my experience. It is the greatest single cause of true ptosis in eye removal surgery. Except for

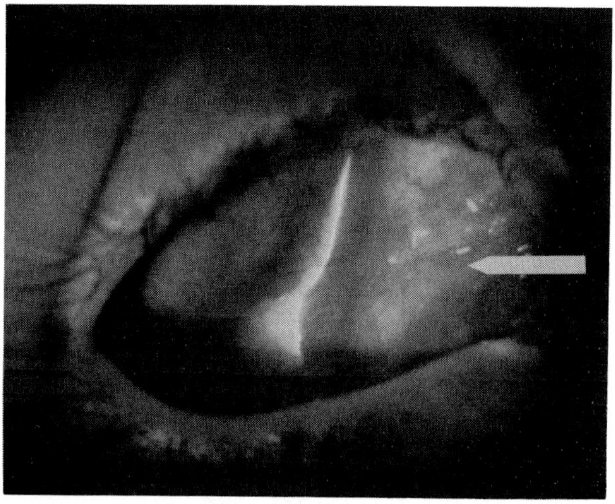

FIG. 18. Slit-lamp photograph of the enucleated OD of a 4-year-old girl in whom the rectus muscles were imbricated over a 16-mm spherical implant in Tenon's capsule. The slit beam, approaching from the right, reveals the superotemporal displacement of the ball and, below it, the retraction of the inferonasally displaced point of imbrication of the rectus muscles.

some rare cases of ptosis which are unexplainable and impossible to correct with prostheses, these ptosis cases are the most difficult to reduce. For these reasons, we should try to understand the cause or causes of the ptosis. I judge that the following two factors contribute to the ptosis:

(a) Upon examining the eye socket after such a surgical procedure, it can be clearly deduced that the point of imbrication of the rectus muscles has slipped off the face of the spherical implant to the lower nasal side (Fig. 18). It slips off in this way because there is a loose expanse of Tenon's capsule present, especially in the superior temporal quadrant between the superior and lateral recti, immediately upon closing Tenon's. There is also a loose bulge in each of the other three quadrants between adjacent rectus muscles, but the large ball cannot easily get into one of these other spaces because of the presence and filling effect of the oblique muscles nasally and the ligament of Lockwood inferiorly.

As the superior rectus slides off the face of the sphere, it tugs on Müller's muscle and the levator (Fig. 19). It seems reasonable to believe that there is damage to the muscles as a result. Even if the muscles are not traumatized to cause the ptosis, the downward tug could pull the levator muscle forward and downward to cause almost equally bad ptosis. The superior nasal fornix is also being pulled downward.

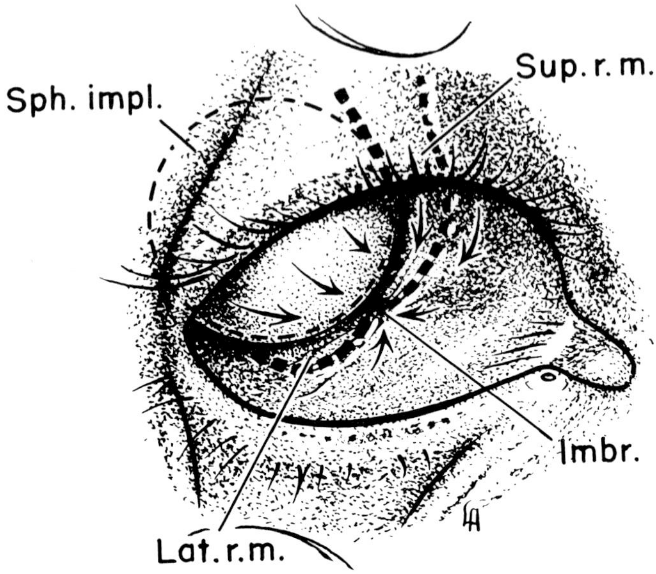

FIG. 19. Schematic drawing, interpreting the typical appearance of the eye socket in enucleation, with rectus muscles imbricated over spherical implants: *Sph. impl.*, spherical implant which has migrated into loose pocket of Tenon's capsule between lateral and superior rectus muscles; *Lat. r. m.*, lateral rectus muscle which has slipped downward and under implant; *Sup. r. m.*, superior rectus muscle which has slipped nasally and nearly behind implant; *Imbr.*, point of imbrication of four rectus muscles, slipped downward nasally and pulled backward under implant; *arrows* indicate displacement by tension of conjunctiva – downward and nasally over implant and centrally from other areas.

(b) As the point of imbrication of the rectus muscles slips downward nasally and backward around the ball, it naturally pulls and stretches the anterior central part of Tenon's capsule down and around with it. Conjunctiva stretches downward nasally with Tenon's. These two structures together can stretch only so far. Beyond that point, there has to be a direct pull upon the superior temporal fornix and all interconnected tissues in the region (Fig. 19). Thus, in turn, the connective tissues related to Müller's muscle and the tarsus are pulled so that the bulbar conjunctiva, superior temporal fornix and upper eyelid all come downward together.

(Imbrication of the four recti over smaller ball implants does not usually cause marked ptosis. However, imbrication usually causes the ball to migrate into one or another of the quadrants. Because the ball is smaller, it can occasionaly be displaced below and temporally, or rarely, even into one of the nasal quadrants. Sockets with such migrated spheres are difficult to fit by the traditional method and should always be fitted on the basis of impressions.)

The danger of migration of spherical implants from under imbricated rectus muscles has been recognized for many years by certain experienced surgeons. In 1938, John Wheeler [15] reported a specially designed hollow glass implant incorporating grooves for the four rectus muscles to prevent displacement. He advocated implantation at a second operation rather than at the time of enucleation. Possibly, this type of implant, made of plastic, might be successful if it were tried again.

The conclusion from the foregoing observations is that the rectus muscles should never be imbricated over the front of any completely spherical ball implant. If a sphere must be used, the type of surgery described by Costen [16] (but with no larger than 18-mm spheres) is recommended. Even this type of surgery does not always prevent displacement of the spheres, but it offers a much more favorable potential.

6. *Enucleation with buried, quasi-integrated muscle cone implant* (My experience has been largely limited to the Allen and Iowa implants [8-10,17].) has frequently been accompanied by very mild ptosis but only rarely by marked ptosis. Failure to adequately free the sheath of the superior rectus muscle during surgery of the Allen or the Iowa implant might cause the levator muscle to be pulled forward to cause mild ptosis. Such amounts may be easily corrected by the complex prosthetic method.

7. *Simple evisceration* is often accompanied by mild to moderate ptosis. The sclera shrinks to a small nubbin in the center of the orbit following this operation. The superior rectus is pulled downward, which then pulls Müller's muscle and the levator muscle downward through the junction of the muscle sheaths, probably thus contributing to the ptosis.

I rarely see simple eviscerations now but those I have seen in the past have not been easy to fit well. Furthermore, statistically, the motility of the prosthesis is not good after this operation. With the rectus muscles lying practically against each other down the center of the orbit, they cannot move tissue near the fornices, as is necessary for imparting good motility to the artificial eye. As far as prosthesis fitting is concerned, this operation should not be used unless the surgeon finds it absolutely necessary.

8. *Evisceration with small intrascleral spherical implants* is little better, as far as ptosis is concerned, than simple evisceration. There can be ptosis, the motility is not particularly good, and these sockets are not particularly easy to fit.

9. *Eviscerations with either excised cornea and 16-mm spherical implant or retained cornea and 18-mm implant* [18,19] are the most

desirable from many standpoints and are least likely of any surgical procedure to cause ptosis. I have not seen obvious ptosis with them and there is no logical reason why the surgery should produce more than the mildest pseudoptosis. Any marked ptosis which may occur will probably be coincidental – from causes other than the surgery.

Flush fitting of cosmetic shells over these implants is preferred and both of these types of surgery are heartily recommended for the benefit of both the patients and the ocularists. However, 20-mm diameter, completely spherical implants should never be used in evisceration. They are too large in the AP diameter to leave room for normal depth of the prosthetic "anterior chamber." Admittedly, this is not noticeable except upon close scrutiny, but the technical problems of coloring and fabricating the prosthetic shell are much greater than with thicker shells over 16- or 18-mm spherical implants.

Summary

The types of ptosis have been grouped and classified in a manner which will be advantageous so far as a prosthetic management of ptosis is concerned.

The methods for reduction or correction of ptosis by size of prosthesis, the use of shelves or crutches and the shaping of plastic eyes have been listed. The rather recently devised, complex method has been outlined in more detail because of its superiority.

The frequency and degree of ptosis related to each different prosthetic situation, from scarred living eyes through simple enucleation to evisceration with large spherical implants, have been estimated on the basis of my own experience. The especially high correlation of severe ptosis with imbrication of the rectus muscles over large spherical implants in Tenon's capsule has been emphasized.

The need for all ocularists to know the anatomy of the orbit and the appropriate related mechanical principles in order to apply the complex method of ptosis reduction has been expressed. I have also expressed my opinion that there must be continuing exchange of knowledge and new information and close cooperation between the ophthalmologist and ocularist in order to progress and to make the best fitting procedures available to patients everywhere.

References

1. Gougelman, Paul: Fitting of prostheses for patients with creptophthalmos and extreme microphthalmos. Arch. Ophthal., 18:774-776, 1937.
2. Gougelmann, Pierre: The fitting of artificial eyes. Arch. Ophthal., 2:76-79, 1929.

3. Beard, C.: Blepharoptosis: Clinical evaluation and therapeutic rationale. *In* Smith, B. and Cherubini, T. D. (eds.): Ophthalmic Plastic Surgery. St. Louis:C. V. Mosby Co., 1970. International Clinics, 10:97-115, 1970.
4. Allen, L., Braley, A. E. and Webster, H.: Problems in ocular prostheses. J. Iowa Med. Soc., 43:329-335, 1953.
5. Allen, L. and Webster, H.: Modified impression method of artificial eye fitting. Amer. J. Ophthal., 67:189-218, 1969.
6. Allen, L.: Fitting the prosthesis: A challenge. Trans. Amer. Acad. Ophthal. Otolaryng., 74:1318-1320, 1970.
7. Allen, L.: Modified impression fitting, *In* Shannon, G. M. and Connelly, F. J. (eds.): Oculoplastic Surgery and Prosthetics. International Clinics, 10:747-762, 1970.
8. Allen, L., Ferguson, E. C., III and Braley, A. E.: A quasi-integrated buried muscle cone implant with good motility and advantages for prosthetic fitting. Trans. Amer. Acad. Ophthal. Otolaryng., 64:272-284, 1960.
9. Spivey, B. E., Allen, L. and Burns, C. A.: The Iowa enucleation implant. A 10-year evaluation of technique and results. Amer. J. Ophthal., 67:171-188, 1969.
10. Allen, L., Spivey, B. E. and Burns, C. A.: A larger Iowa implant. Amer. J. Ophthal., 68:397-400, 1969.
11. Heyman, L. S.: Prosthetic aids in blepharoptosis: Shelf devices. *In* Shannon, G. M. and Connelly, F. G. (eds.): Ophthalmic Plastic Surgery and Prosthetics. International Clinics, vol 10, 1970.
12. LeGrand, J. A.: Scleral cosmetic shells and lenses. *In* Shannon, G. M. and Connelly, F. G. (eds.): Surgery and Prosthetics. International Clinics, 10:763-776, 1970.
13. Jahrling, R. C.: Prosthetics for upper lid deformities. *In* Shannon, G. M. and connelly, F. J. (eds.): Oculoplastic Surgery and Prosthetics. International Clinics, vol. 10, 1970.
14. Heyman, L. S.: Ptosis crutch, scleral contact lenses. *In* Girard, L. J. (ed.): St. Louis:C. V. Mosby, 1967.
15. Wheeler, J. M.: Implantation of hollow grooved body into orbit after enucleation. Arch. Ophthal., 20:709-712, 1938.
16. Costen, T. O.: The spherical implant. Trans. Amer. Acad. Ophthal. Otolaryng., 74:1284-1286, 1950.
17. Allen, J. H. and Allen, L.: A buried muscle cone implant; Development of a tunneled hemispherical type. Arch. Ophthal., 43:879-890, 1950.
18. Mules, P. H.: Evisceration of the globe, with artificial vitreous. Trans. Ophthal. Soc. U. K., 5:200, 1884-1885.
19. Burch, F. E.: Evisceration of the globe with scleral implant and preservation of the cornea. Trans. Amer. Ophthal. Soc., 34:272-282, 1939; Amer. J. Ophthal., 23:47-51, Jan. 1940.
20. Hughes, W. L.: Evisceration. Arch. Ophthal., 63:36-40, Jan. 1960.
21. Ruedemann, A. D., Jr.: Modified Burch type evisceration with scleral implant. Amer. J. Ophthal., 49:41-54, Jan. 1960.

Surgical Correction of Anophthalmic Upper Lid Ptosis

Richard R. Tenzel, M.D.

If a person has an artificial eye, one might think that he would not need the lid to open and close on the prosthesis; but without a working lid that closes, the patient gets heavy mucus formation and crusting on the prosthesis.

To judge the amount of ptosis present, compare the good eye to the ptotic eye by measuring the palpebral fissure. Levator function is measured with the eye looking down vs. looking far up. The excursion of the lid is called the levator function. These measurements are used in the selection of a surgical procedure for ptosis. *If the ptosis cannot be corrected by an ocularist, then is the time for surgery and only then.* Most of the good fitters can correct 90% of the ptosis present with the anophthalmic eye. Most of the procedures which can be done for a regular ptosis can also be done without an eye present. The anterior route of resection of the levator, as well as the conjunctival route, can be used. A full-thickness excision technique can also be used: make an incision from the skin through to the conjunctival surface, take out a full-thickness section of lid (almost millimeter for millimeter for the amount to be corrected), and simply close the defect. On downgaze and also in attempts at closure, however, these lids just do not close well. Therefore, I do not believe this is the procedure of choice.

A procedure recently advocated by Dr. Lester Jones and popularized by the late Dr. Marvin Quickert is the repair of the dehiscence of the levator aponeurosis. I use it in anophthalmic ptosis, but I call it a levator plication. This is not my technique or procedure, but I think it works well. There is not much of a lid lag with this procedure because there is little shortening of the aponeurosis.

Richard R. Tenzel, M.D., Clinical Associate Professor of Ophthalmology, University of Miami School of Medicine; Chief, Ophthalmic Plastic Surgical Service, Bascom Palmer Eye Institute, Miami, Fla.

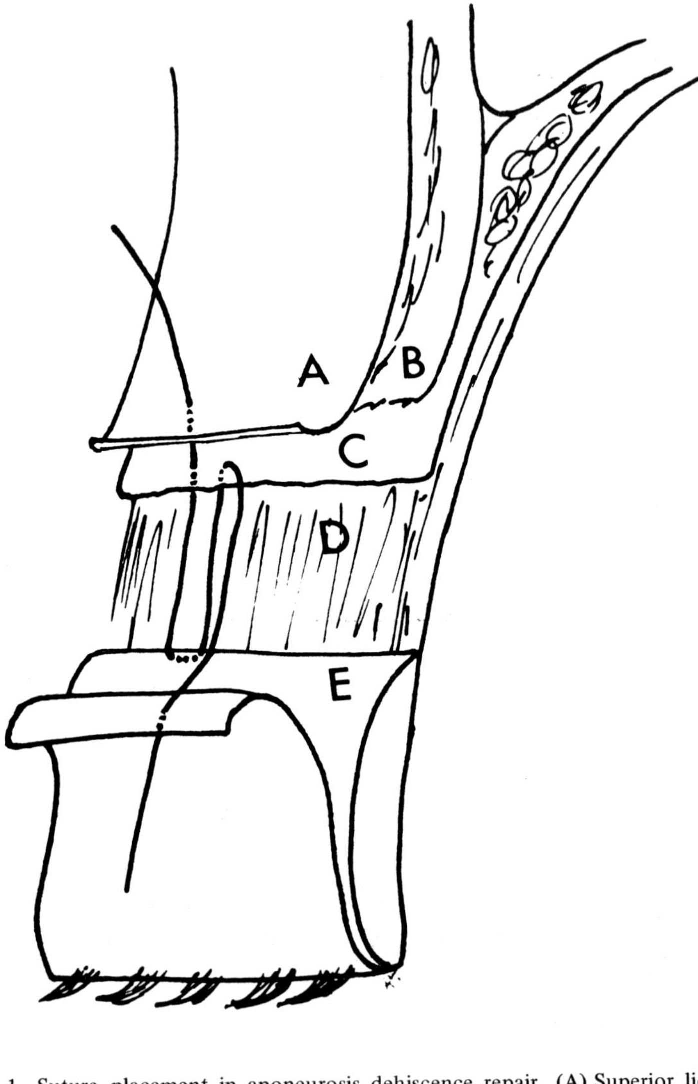

FIG. 1. Suture placement in aponeurosis dehiscence repair. (A) Superior lid skin. (B) Cut orbital septum. (C) Levator aponeurosis. (D) Müller's muscle. (E) Tarsus. The suture goes through upper skin edge, levator aponeurosis, tarsus, back through aponeurosis and out through lower skin edge. (From Tenzel, R. R.: Surgical judgment in ptosis repair. Trans. Amer. Acad. Ophthal. Otolaryng. In press.)

I used to use nonabsorbable sutures but had a problem with small suture granulomas that had to be opened. At the present time, I use one of the polyglycolic acid sutures (Dexon®) as a suture tied on the skin that will absorb and drop out.

The technique is simple. The lid fold is measured on the normal side and a line is made on the ptotic side. A very small amount of anesthetic is used, about 0.50-0.75 cc, injected just beneath the skin line. (You do not want to paralyze the lid because you want to check the elevation of the lid on the table). The incision is made through the skin. The orbicularis muscle is opened to show the orbital septum. The orbital septum is buttonholed; a muscle hook is placed in the septum and one cuts between the skin and the septum to open it across the lid. A nice, glistening aponeurosis is always present beneath the insertion of the orbital septum on the aponeurosis.

I usually take a strip of orbicularis beneath the lower skin flap in order to get a better lid fold. My suture technique (Fig. 1) is really the only thing that is different. It shortens the operation because it is one set of sutures instead of two. The suture goes through the upper skin edge and takes a bite in the levator aponeurosis right where the septum inserted. It then takes a horizontal bite in the tarsus and comes back up through the aponeurosis, making a horizontal mattress suture in the levator aponeurosis. The suture comes out through the lower skin edge. This makes the upper skin bite at a different plane than the lower skin bite; so they are slightly separated. This allows the lid to twist into the wound and gives a good lid fold. The patient is able to open and close his eye, and one can titrate the procedure while he is still on the operating table.

Lowering the Upper Lid Level with a Prosthesis

Raymond A. Rarey

Many sockets are seen with lids too wide open, even without a conformer or prosthesis in place. This is especially true with simple evisceration and simple enucleation.

It is the duty of the ocularist to correct this problem whenever possible. Illustrated are four mechanical principles used separately or in combination to correct the problem.

Figure 1A shows a cross section of a wax pattern before any attempt has been made to lower the lid. In Figure 1B the iris-cornea piece is set back several millimeters to recess the front surface; this must not be overdone as it will give too flat an appearance to the prosthesis.

Figure 2A shows the set-back iris-cornea piece before reshaping the wax. Figure 2B is the recontoured wax pattern.

In Figure 3 wax is added to the upper section of the pattern to straighten the vertical plane. The added wax is much thicker at the top; as a result the tarsal plate will be tilted forward and the lid margin will move downward.

In Figure 4 several millimeters have been removed from the superior section of the wax pattern to lessen the amount of support on the levator muscle and surrounding tissues, allowing the lid to drop down.

The complete mechanical procedures used to lower the upper lid are shown in Figure 5.

Cosmetic optics will be of aid in correcting any small amount of defect not accomplished by the four preceding techniques. When the prosthesis is made much thinner than usual to allow the lid to close more, and the eyelids are recessed and the lids are still too wide open, glasses with a

---

Raymond A. Rarey, Certified Ocularist, Department of Ophthalmology, University Hospitals, Iowa City, Iowa.

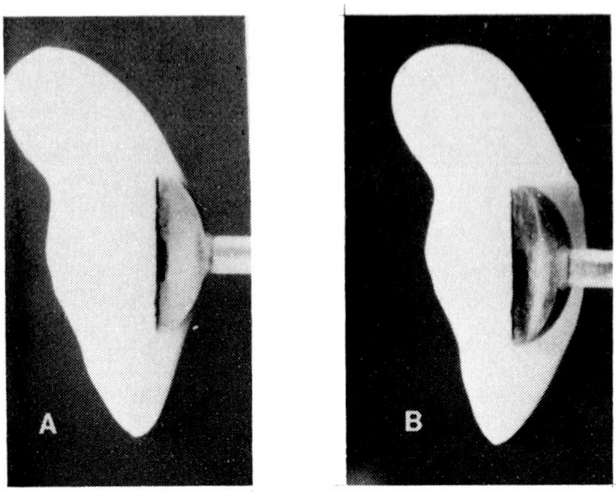

FIGURE 1.

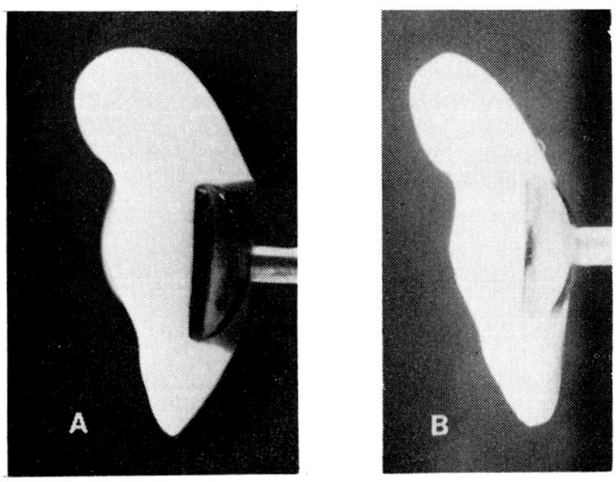

FIGURE 2.

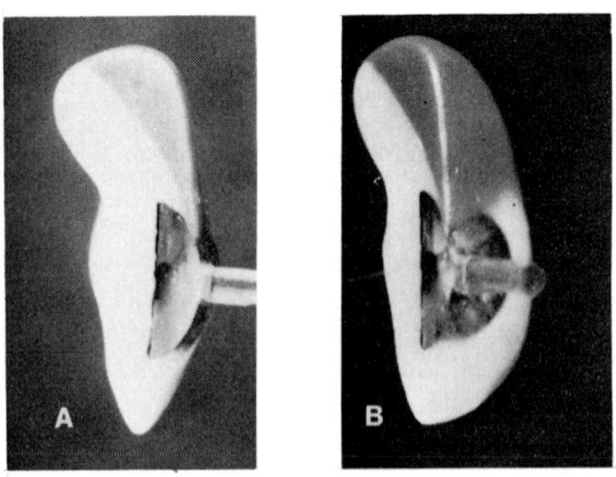

FIGURE 3.

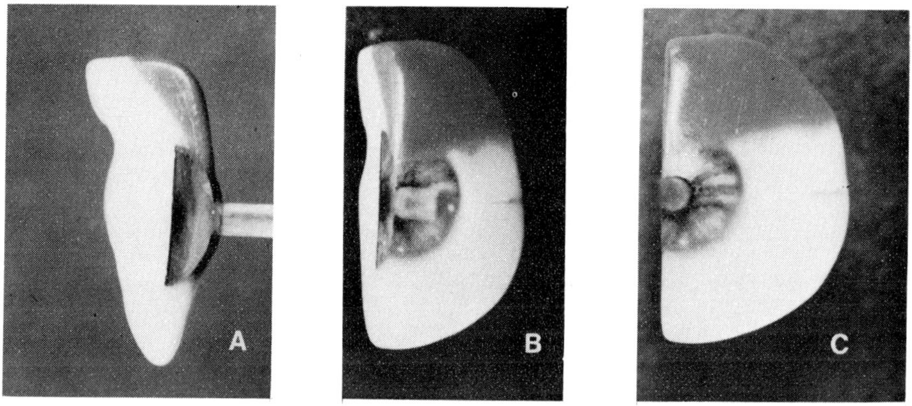

FIGURE 4.

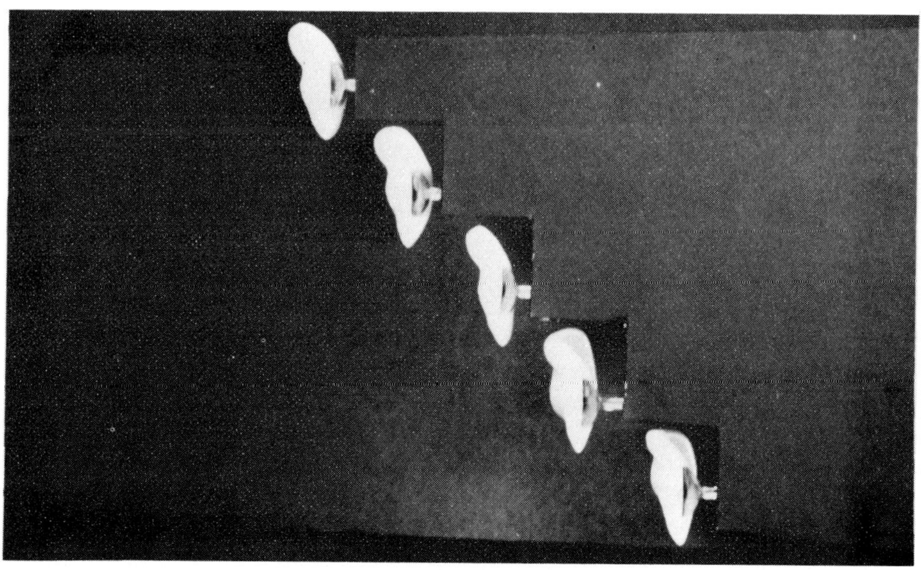

FIGURE 5.

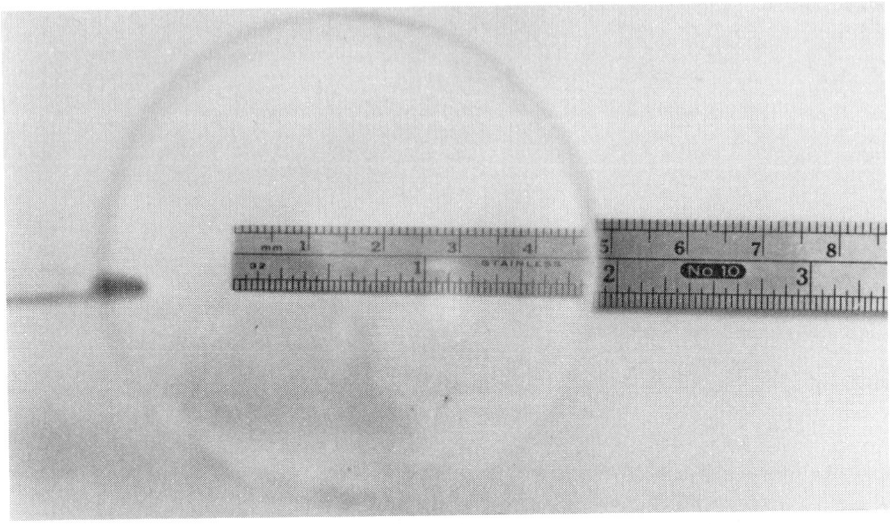

FIGURE 6.

minus-sphere lens on the prosthetic side will minify the image to make the lids appear more closed (Fig. 6). With the minus lens the image of the eye and eyelids will be shifted toward the lens and counteract much of the recessed appearance.

Influence and Correction of Anophthalmic Entropion and Ectropion by Prostheses

David Bulgarelli

Problems in fitting ophthalmic prosthetics include entropion, ectropion and sagging of the lower eyelid. The ocularist can sometimes bring the lower eyelid well toward the required condition or correct the defect without the patient undergoing surgery, by physically manipulating the tarsal plate and other tissues of the lower eyelid with the shape of the prosthesis.

Entropion, inversion of the eyelid margin, can be caused by any of the following factors: (a) contraction of scar tissue in the palpebral conjunctiva or underlying tarsus, (b) a combination of tonic spasm of the orbicularis muscle and laxity of tissues in the lower eyelid, (c) orbital fractures, (d) severe crushing injuries [1], (e) changes caused by alkali, acid and thermal burns, (f) multiple orbital surgery, (g) implant extrusion, (h) orbital shrinkage due to chronic infection of the eye socket [1], (i) prolonged absence of a prosthesis [2], or (j) extended wearing of an ill-fitting prosthesis. Also, where an entropion is not evident but the tissue changes are already present, the insertion of a prosthesis not designed for correction will divulge the defect.

The method used in shaping the prosthesis to influence the shape of the lower eyelid and eyelashes (Fig. 1B and C) is to reverse the curvature of the anterior surface of the prosthesis, starting slightly superior to the desired level of the eyelid margin (*b*) and coming to a more vertical plane at the bottom edge, thus forming a trough-like surface across the anteroinferior surface from the medial to the temporal canthus [3]. If the eyelid is flexible enough to follow the recurved surface of the prosthesis, and if there is enough conjunctiva, the tarsal plate of the lower eyelid and

---

David Bulgarelli, Department of Ophthalmology, University of Iowa College of Medicine, Iowa City.

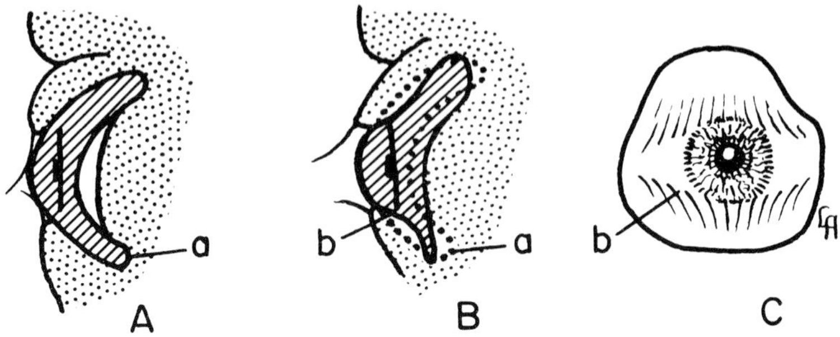

FIG. 1. Entropion. (A) Cross section; Snellen reform prosthesis shape opposite of that needed for correction, eyelashes lying on prosthesis cornea. (B) Cross section; dotted outline is the shape of Snellen reform prosthesis in (A); shaded area shows changes of shape to reduce entropion. (C) Front view of same changes as in (B) (see text).

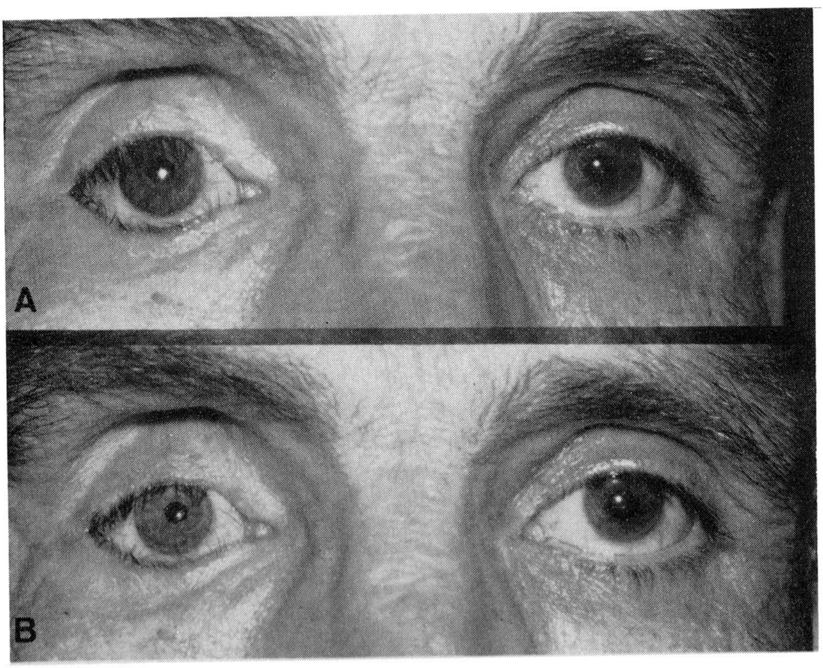

FIG. 2. Entropion, right eye. (A) Snellen reform prosthesis, eyelashes touching prosthesis. (B) Prosthesis of corrected shape, eyelashes raised slightly off prosthesis.

the eyelashes will be turned forward in a more acceptable physiologic and cosmetic direction. But, depending on the cause and amount of the entropion, the lower eyelid conjunctiva and the tarsal plate may not follow the shape of the prosthesis and a minimal correction will be obtained.

The ocularist can only correct the mild cases of entropion. (Figs. 2 and 3). This 48-year-old man had late complications following enucleation, with orbital scarring causing an entropion of the eyelids. The prosthesis was fitted, giving enough correction to decrease the previous amount of irritation (Figs. 2B and 3B).

The usual complication with entropion is continual mucoid discharge caused by the constant irritation of the eyelashes turning inward and the typical failure of closure of the eyelids. When this is present, there is little that the ocularist can do to improve the situation for the patient, and if any improvement is desired, or can be expected, the attention of an ophthalmologist is required.

Ectropion, eversion of the eyelid margin, exposes an excessive amount of palpebral conjunctiva and scleral portion of the prosthesis [4]. It can be a result of contraction of scar tissue in the lid or contraction of the skin; reduced tonus of the orbicularis muscle; paralysis of the facial nerve which

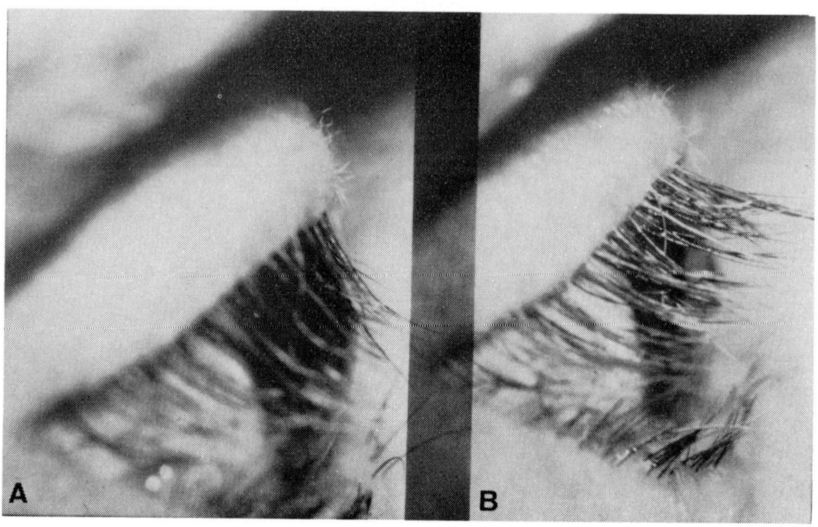

FIG. 3. Side view, (A) and (B) coinciding with (A) and (B) of Figure 2.

causes loss of the contractile power of the orbicularis muscle; chronic thickening of the palpebral portion of the muscle; senility; atrophic changes in the skin; herniation of fat into the lower fornix area due to weakness of, or damage to, the ligament of Lockwood; migration of an orbital implant into the lower cul-de-sac [5, 6]; weakness of all connective tissue; and external thermal and chemical burns [7] in which lid tissue and skin sustain the major injury.

When an ophthalmic prosthesis is fitted where ectropion is present, there are usually secondary changes such as foreshortened inferior cul-de-sac and/or lower eyelid sag. In fact, if the prosthesis is not correctly fitted, it can exaggerate the amount of ectropion and sagging of the lower eyelid enough to seriously affect retention of the prosthesis (Fig. 4A). There can be poor retention to complete failure of retention of the prosthesis in the eye socket by eversion of the tarsal plate and, thus, the lower lid, allowing the rounded lower edge of the prosthesis to slip out.

The patient shown in Figure 4 sustained injuries from grenade shrapnel in Viet Nam. He was referred to our clinic because of poor retention of the prosthesis and continual mucoid discharge. A new prosthesis was com-

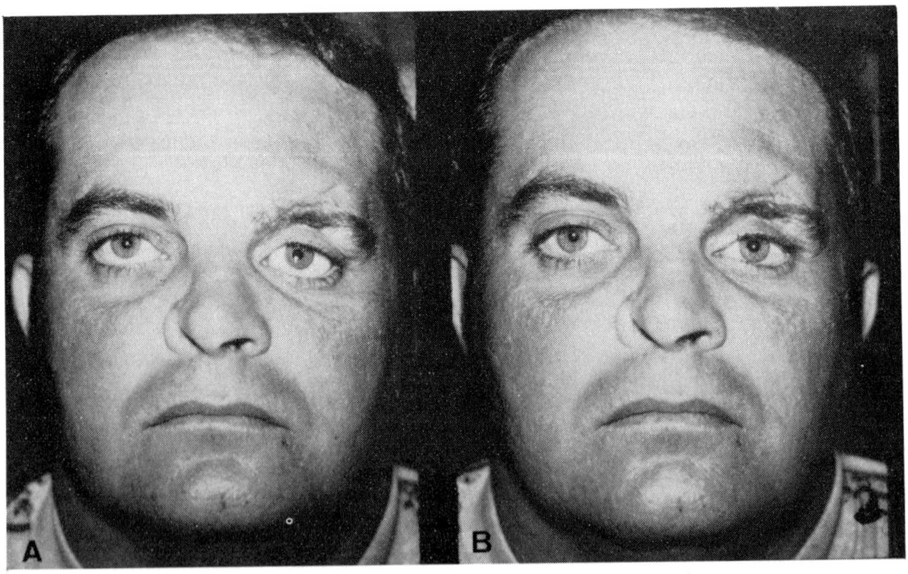

FIG. 4. (A) Ectropion, sagging left lower eyelid and poor retention of prosthesis with reform-shaped artificial eye. (B) Corrected shape reducing lower eyelid ectropion and improving retention of prosthesis.

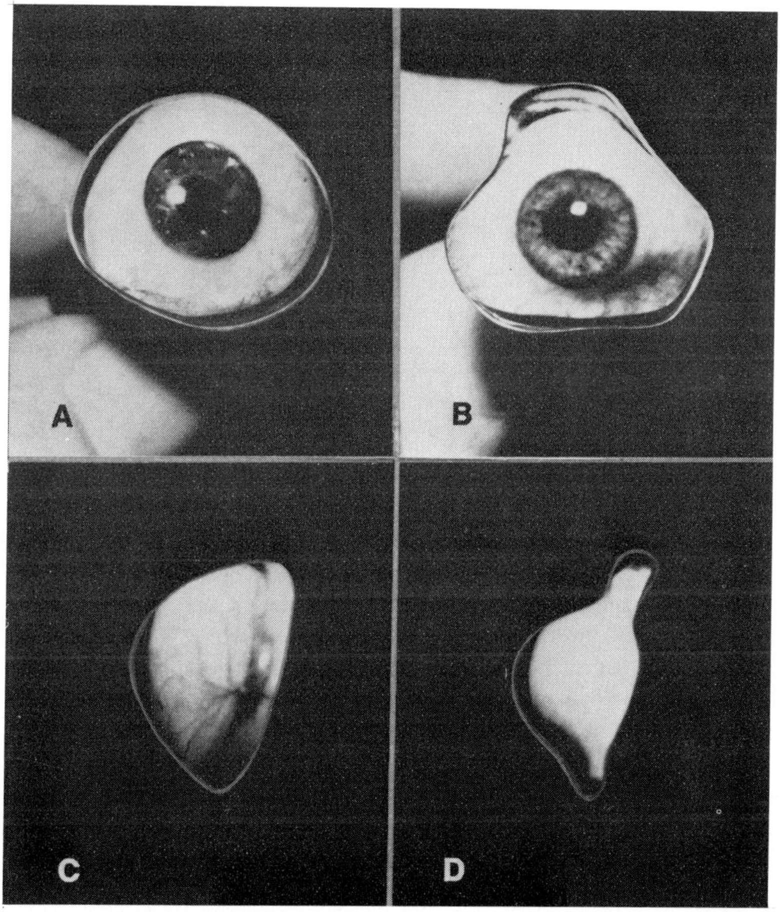

FIG. 5. Front (A and B) and side (C and D) views of prostheses shown in (A) and (B), respectively, of Figure 4.

pleted (Fig. 4B). After his lower eyelid was raised to the desired height by applying the appropriate mechanical principles in the fitting, it was necessary to use the ptosis modifications to raise his upper eyelid, as described by Allen and Webster [3]. Front and side views of the prostheses show the form modifications (Fig. 5).

Modifying the prosthesis for an effective correction of ectropion can be accomplished by substituting a longer, thinner, more vertical lower portion (*b*) (Figs. 6B and C) for the former shape at (*a*) (Figs. 6A and B)[3]. This lower portion can be less than 1 mm thick if necessary, as long

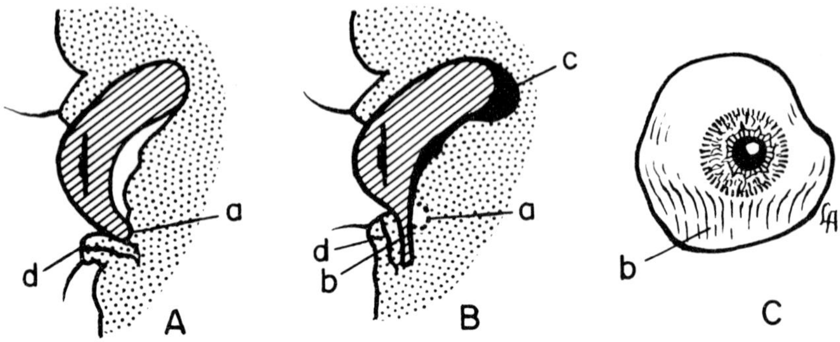

FIG. 6. Form modification for ectropion. (A) Cross section of Snellen reform-shaped prosthesis and uncorrected ectropion of lower eyelid. (B) Cross section; dotted outline (*a*) was shape of lower edge of prosthesis in (A); solid line (*b*) is corrected shape of lower edge to reduce ectropion; black area (*c*) represents changes in the prosthesis to conform to an impression of the socket tissues and to keep the eye in an upright position. (C) Front view showing form modifications (see text).

as the very edge is well rounded and polished. This thin, rather flat extension often presses easily downward to rotate the lower tarsus (*d*) from a relatively horizontal plane in (A) to a more vertical plane in (B). Any tendency for the prosthesis to tilt backward gives the lower edge a start toward slipping over the lower eyelid. When necessary, material (*c*) should be added along the back of the top edge of the wax pattern to keep it propped in an upright position. This serves in exactly the same way and as effectively as the "hook" added for this purpose at the back of the traditional prosthesis, but with more comfort for the patient. This same form modification which corrects the ectropion will improve the retention of the prosthesis.

The eye of the 64-year-old man shown in Figure 7 was enucleated due to absolute glaucoma and retinal vein occlusion. There were no complications during the surgery or postoperatively. When the patient came for the prosthesis fitting, marked ectropion was present (Fig. 7B). Figure 7C shows the final prosthesis in place. The shape of the prosthesis was similar to that shown in Figure 6.

The complications seem to be few with ectropion. When the defect is extreme, it may not be possible to turn the lower eyelid inward enough so that the nasal punctum contacts the prosthesis, thus preventing pooling and overflow of tears and contributing to their proper removal into the efferent portion of the lacrimal system. Another complication is the total loss of the lower cul-de-sac with attendant lack of mechanical support

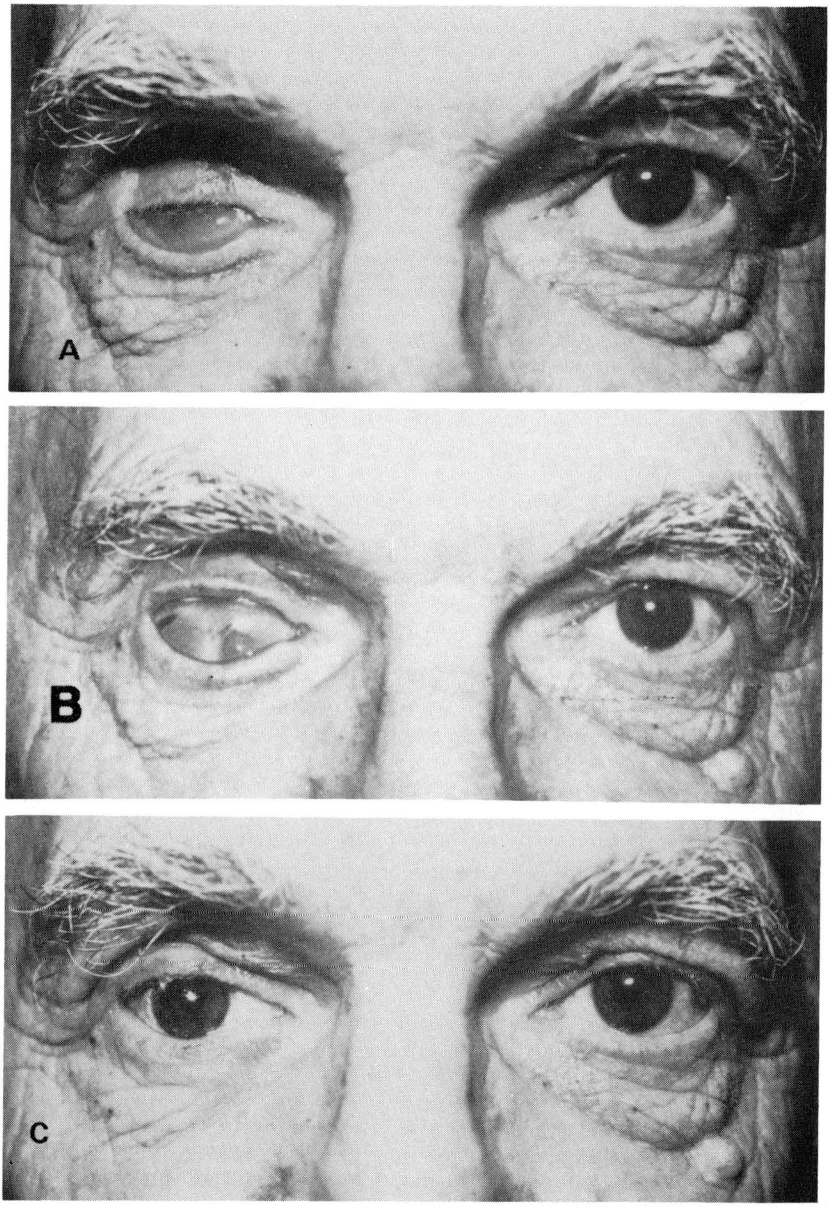

FIG. 7. (A) Ectropion of lower right eyelid without conformer. (B) Same patient with conformer. (C) Prosthesis of corrected shape fully correcting ectropion of lower eyelid.

toward adequate retention of the prosthesis. When the defect is extreme the patient must be referred back to the surgeon.

The problem of entropion can be present but not apparent at the beginning of the prosthesis fitting. This is usually due to the fact that there are no tensions present in the socket without a prosthesis, but the conjunctiva is nevertheless taut. As soon as a prosthesis is introduced, it causes the lid margin and eyelashes to turn inward. The worse the entropion, the more difficult is the correction by prosthesis. The ocularist can only correct the mild cases.

Ectropion of the lower eyelid usually can be corrected. The lower eyelid margin is seldom depressed to any extent by these modifications. If it is, the form modifications for correcting sagging lower eyelids are applied.

References

1. Guibor, P.: Contracted sockets – Statement of problems and treatment. *In* Guibor, P. and Gouglemann, H. P. (eds.): Problems and Treatment of Contracted Sockets, Exenterated Orbits and Alkali Burns. Miami:Symposia Specialists, 1973.
2. Kelly, J.: Contraction of the anophthalmic orbit – Statement of the problem and prosthetic treatment. *In* Guibor, P. and Gouglemann, H. P. (eds): Problems and Treatment of Contracted Sockets, Exenterated Orbits and Alkali Burns. Miami: Symposia Specialists, 1973.
3. Allen, L. and Webster, H.: Modified impression method of artificial eye fitting. Amer. J. Ophthal., 67 (2):3, 1969.
4. Prince, J. H.: Recent Advances in Ocular Prosthetics. Edinburgh:E. & S. Livingstone Ltd., 1950.
5. Siliquini, J.: Migration and extrusion of the implant. *In* Shannon, G. M. and Connelly, F. J. (eds.): Oculoplastic Surgery and Prosthetics, International Clinics, vol. 10, no. 4, 1970.
6. Lewis, F.: Migration of ocular implants. *In* Shannon, G. M. and Connelly, F. J. (eds.): Oculoplastic Surgery and Prosthetics, International Clincs, vol. 10, no. 4, 1970.
7. Mulberger, R.: Trauma with lid deformities. *In* Shannon, G. M. and Connelly, F. J. (eds.): Oculoplastic Surgery and Prosthetics, International Clinics, vol. 10, no. 4, 1970.

Surgical Correction of Anophthalmic Entropion and Ectropion of the Lower Lid

Merrill J. Reeh, M.D. and Charles K. Beyer, M.D.

Malpositions of the lower eyelid may produce a cosmetic blemish, lead to inflammation or result in a socket which cannot accept or maintain an artificial eye. The margin or the entire lid may turn in or out. In addition, the lower fornix may be partially or completely obliterated, thus complicating the surgical repair. In all cases one desires to maintain the previous normal relationship of the lid to the globe (Fig. 1).

Entropion

Entropion is painless due to the absence of the eye but still distressful to the patient because the lashes ride on the artificial eye, producing an unsightly appearance by gathering mucus and debris. In severe cases the wearing of an artificial eye may be impossible until this defect is corrected (Fig. 2).

Senile entropion, which Lester Jones and I believe to be due to degeneration of the aponeurosis (lid retractor), may be a problem in the anophthalmic case. We believe this type of entropion results from an inadequate retractor. Because of this the lid is not kept in its proper position. The lid also fails to move properly when the patient looks down. In addition to the loose, stretched retractor, one finds degenerated skin, looseness of the preseptal muscle and mild recession of the globe due to atrophy of the orbital fat. The preseptal muscle moves upward onto the tarsus and pretarsal muscle, and aids in the turning in of a lid which is not adequately maintained by its retractor (Fig. 3).

Merrill J. Reeh, M.D., Chief, Ophthalmic Plastic Surgery Section, Devers Memorial Eye Clinic, Portland, Ore. and Charles K. Beyer, M.D., Director, Department of Ophthalmic Plastic Surgery, Massachusetts Eye and Ear Infirmary, Boston.

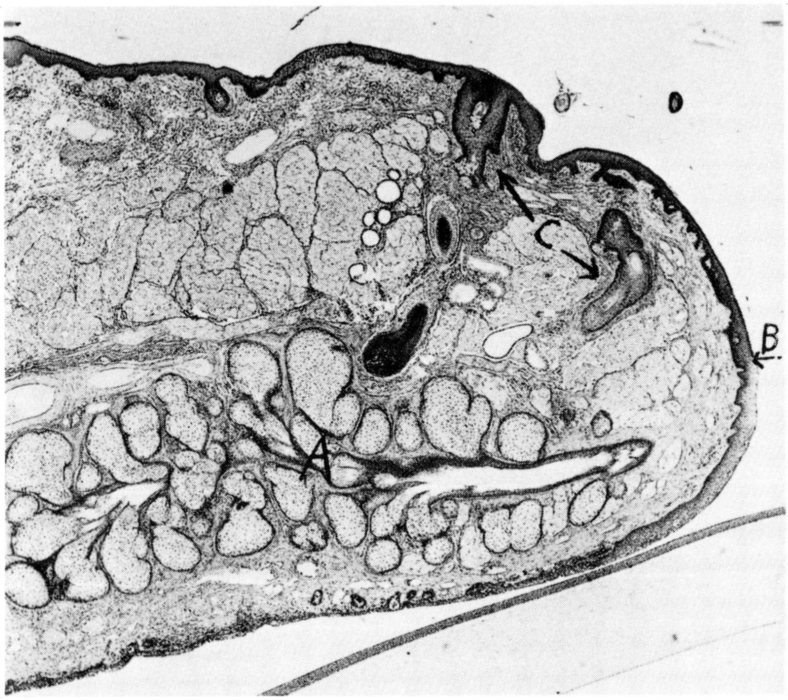

FIG. 1. Normal relationship of lower eyelid to the globe. (A) Meibomian gland. (B) Mucocutaneous junction, "gray line." (C) Hair follicles with associated Zeis and Moll glands.

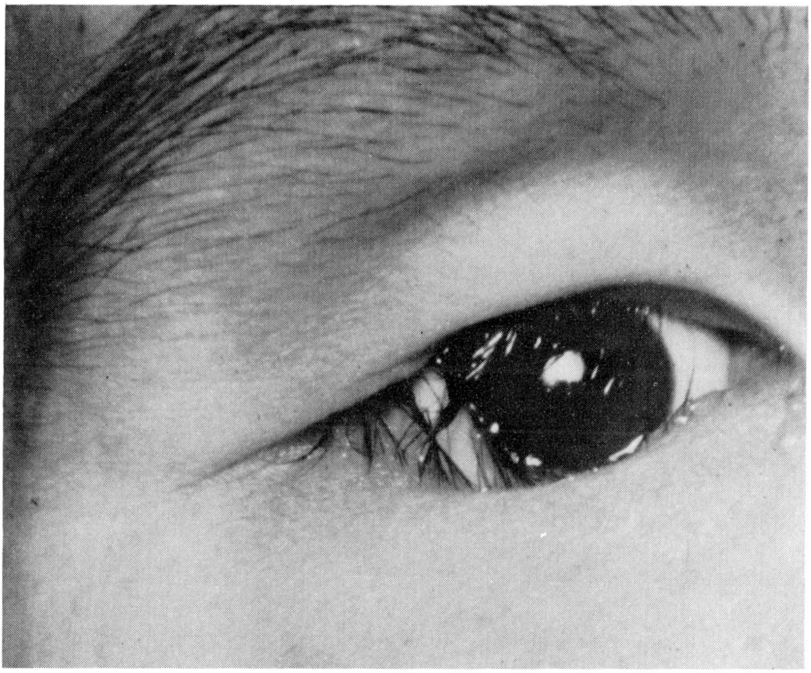

FIG. 2. Severe entropion causing lashes to ride on the artificial eye.

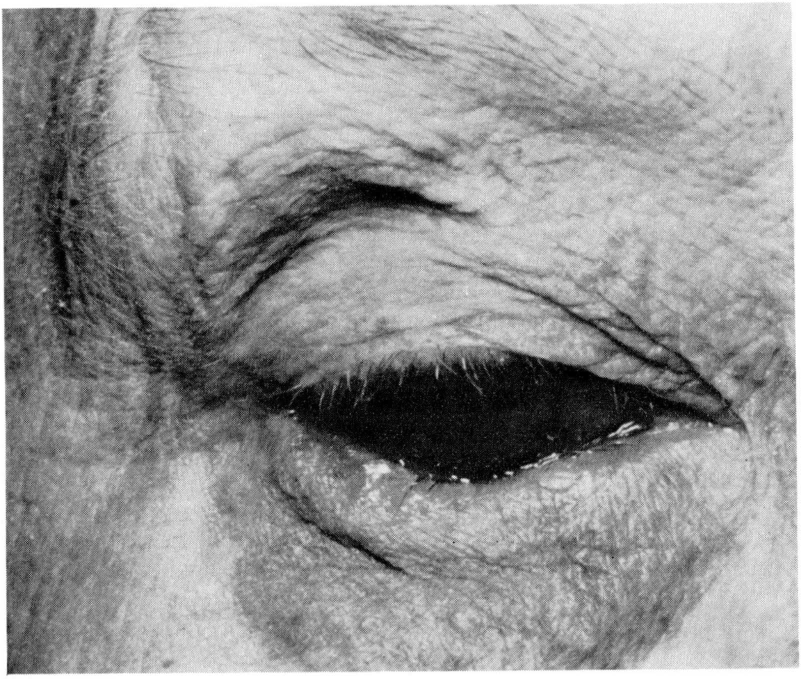

FIG. 3. Senile entropion of the lower lid.

Many procedures have been devised to correct senile entropion. In 1948 Butler devised an operation which altered the tarsus. He resected a wedge of tarsus, placing the apex at the lid margin. This brought the tarsus snugly against the globe, thus discouraging further turning in. This simple procedure is still useful, especially in correcting senile entropion associated with anophthalmos. There have been a number of modifications made by other surgeons during the intervening years.

In more severe cases the procedure developed by Jones and Reeh, and later reported with modifications by Jones, Reeh and Wobig, has proven highly satisfactory. In this operation the retractor (aponeurosis) is shortened by folding much like the closure of an accordion. The same sutures which produce the folding effect close the skin in such a manner to produce a scar barrier that prevents the future overriding of the preseptal muscle on the tarsus. It then exercises its normal function as an elevator of the lower lid. A modest resection of redundant skin may be necessary (Figs. 4 and 5). Cicatricial entropian usually results from chronic inflammatory conditions like trachoma, pemphigoid and Stevens-Johnson syndrome. Burns, trauma and surgical wounds may also cause entropion. In addition to the entropion, the lower fornix may be deficient. Attempts to force into the socket an adequate-sized artificial eye result in an eye which stares and has unsightly debris on the lashes. Both must be corrected before an eye can be worn with satisfaction.

Numerous modifications have been made of the Weiss operation to correct cicatricial entropion. Beyer has developed a procedure which is relatively simple to perform and, if executed properly, usually succeeds in everting the lid margin permanently (Fig. 6).

Lower Fornix

Deficiency of the lower fornix may exist alone or in association with entropion, ectropion or sagging of the lower lid. It varies in severity, depending upon the amount of scar tissue and contracture of the conjunctiva. If it is not too severe and sufficient conjunctiva is present, the fornix can be re-formed without the use of a graft. A small opening is made near the lateral end of the lower fornix. A small scissors is introduced and, with sharp and blunt dissection, the conjunctiva is well freed for the entire length of the fornix. After it is freed adequately to permit re-formation of a deeper fornix, five double-armed, 4-0 silk sutures are looped over a small silicone rod, passed downward through the tissues to emerge through the skin above the margin of the orbit. They are drawn down, causing the sulcus to be formed. Each is tied over a cotton bolster

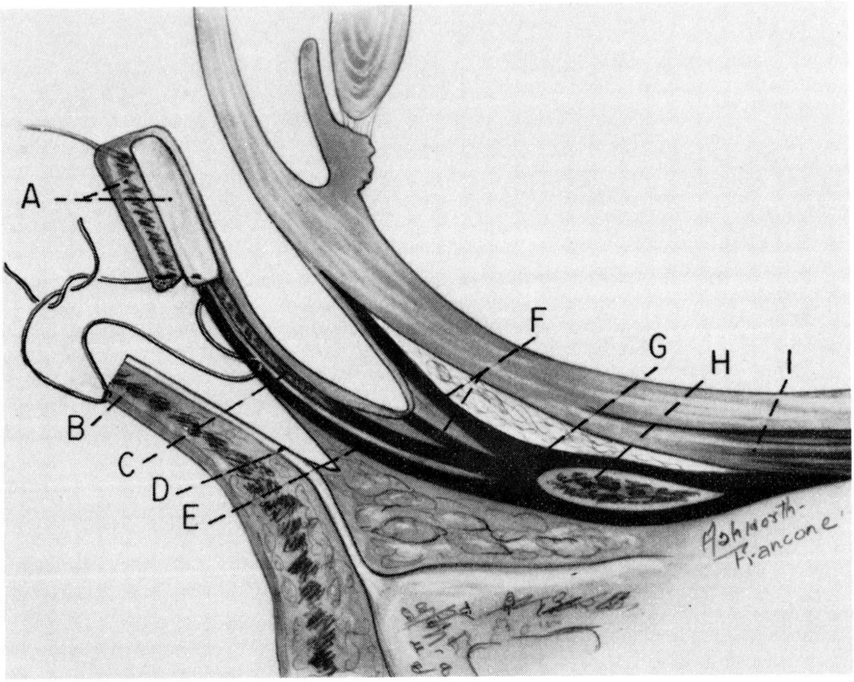

FIG. 4. Cross section diagram. (A) Tarsus, pretarsal skin and muscle. (B) Preseptal skin and muscle. (C) Inferior tarsal muscle (Müller's). (D) Septum orbitale. (E) Aponeurosis of the capsulopalpebral head of the inferior rectus muscle. (F) Tenon's capsule and fascia attaching to the conjunctival fornix. (G) Inferior transverse ligament (Lockwood). (H) Inferior oblique muscle. (I) Inferior rectus muscle. (Courtesy Jones, Reeh and Wobig: Senile entropion. Amer J. Ophthal., 74:327, Aug. 1972.)

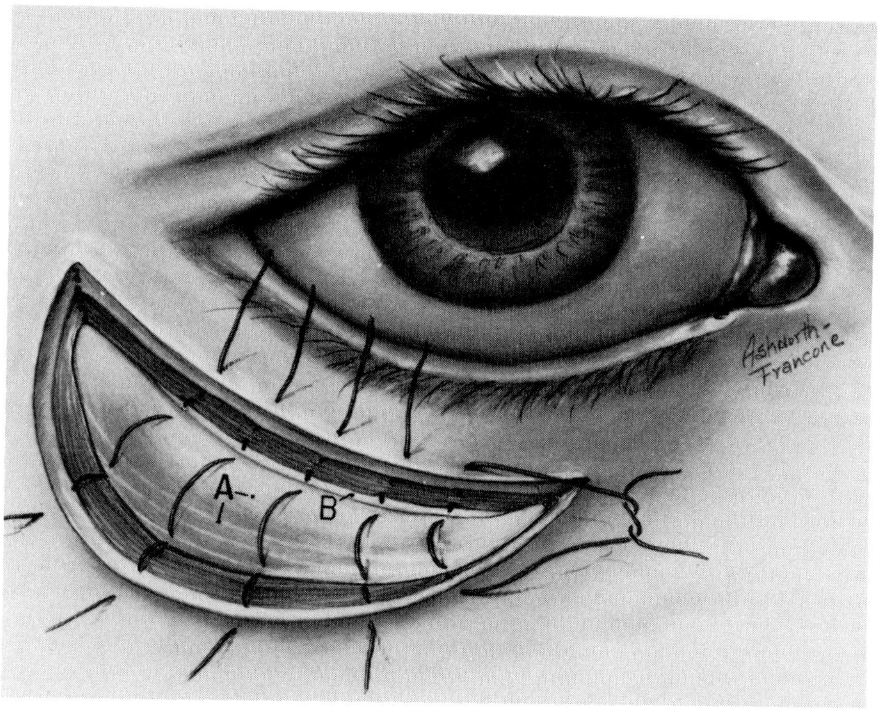

FIG. 5. Frontal diagram. (A) Aponeurosis showing white transverse bands. (B) Lower margin of inferior tarsus. Placement of sutures to produce folding. (Courtesy Jones, Reeh and Wobig: Senile entropion. Amer. J. Ophthal., 74:327, Aug. 1972.)

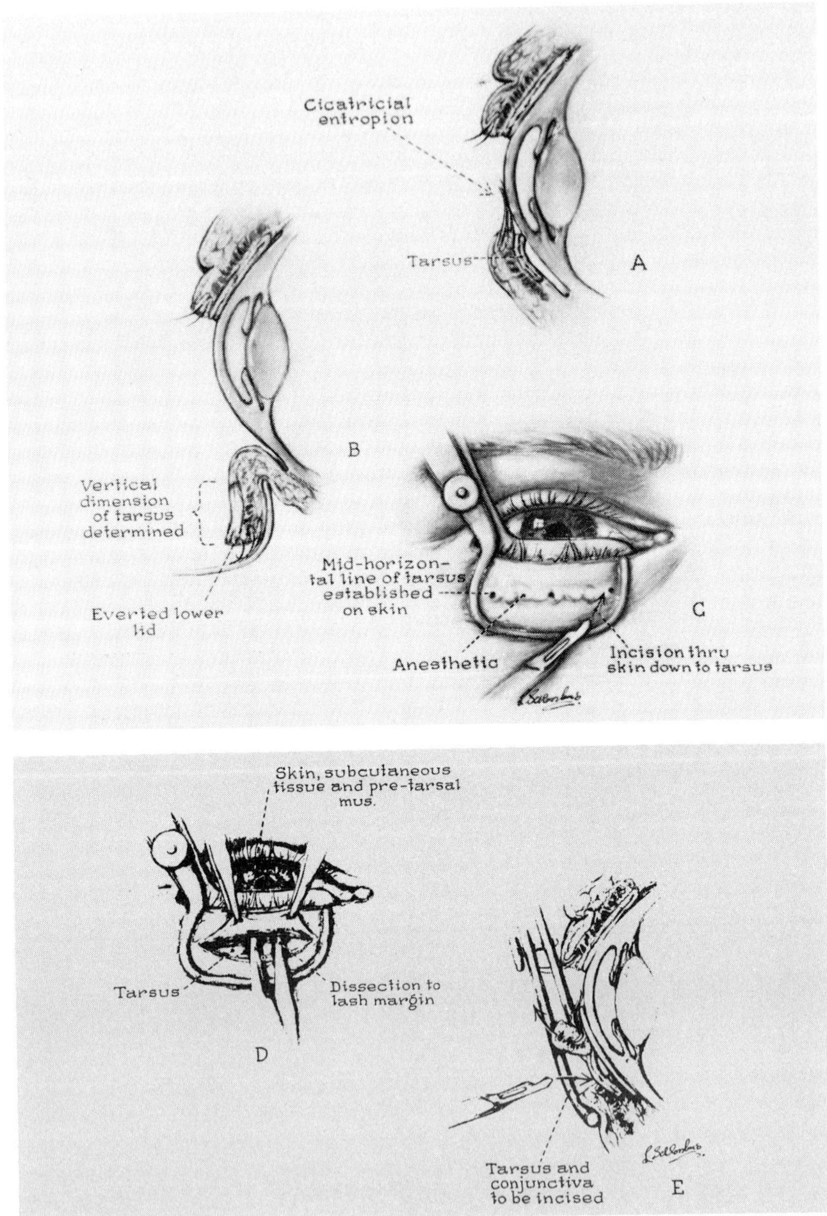

FIG. 6. (A) Schematic appearance of a cicatricial entropion of lower lid. (B through J) Stepwise progression of surgical procedure. (Courtesy Beyer and Carroll: Moderately severe cicatricial entropion. Arch. Ophthal., 89:33, Jan. 1973.)

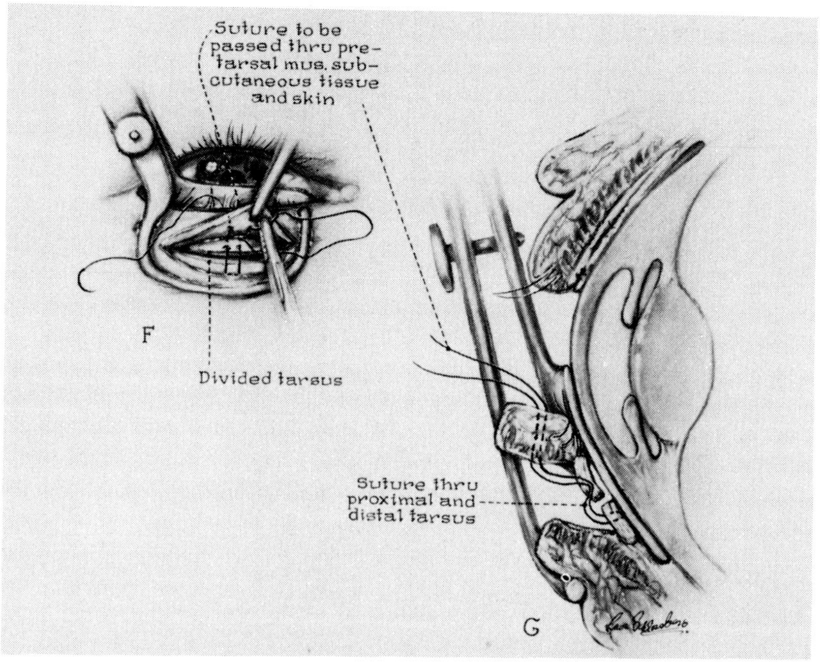
Suture to be passed thru pre-tarsal mus. sub-cutaneous tissue and skin
F
Divided tarsus
Suture thru proximal and distal tarsus
G

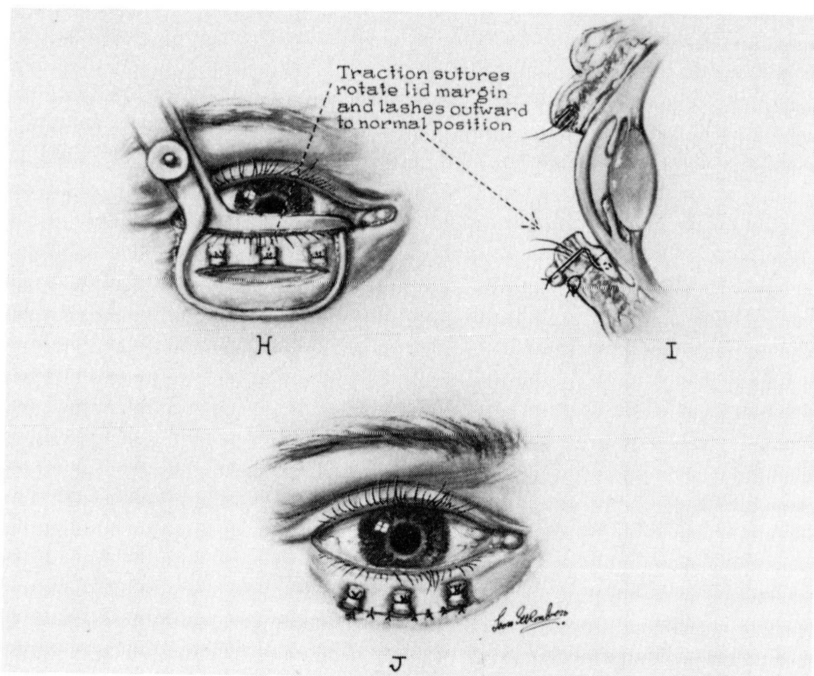
Traction sutures rotate lid margin and lashes outward to normal position
H
I
J

(Figs. 7 and 8). One may combine some procedures to correct a lid malposition with this procedure.

If this defect is more severe, usually with heavy scar and deficient conjunctiva in the fornix, one must excise the scar and replace conjunctiva with an oral mucous membrane graft (Fig. 9). The scar tissue is carefully and meticulously excised and *all* bleeding stopped. A suitable oral mucous membrane graft, 0.4 mm thick, is removed from the lip with a mucotome. When removing a graft it is well to "balloon up" the tissues with physiologic saline before engaging the mucotome. This facilitates better removal of the graft. A suture should be applied immediately in order to identify the mucosal surface, thus preventing the inadvertent suturing of the graft with the wrong surface toward the bed. The graft is sutured carefully into position. I prefer 6-0 chromic gut, interrupted and continuous sutures. When the graft is in place the cleft is established with 4-0 silk sutures looped around a silicone rod to emerge just above the orbital rim (Fig. 10).

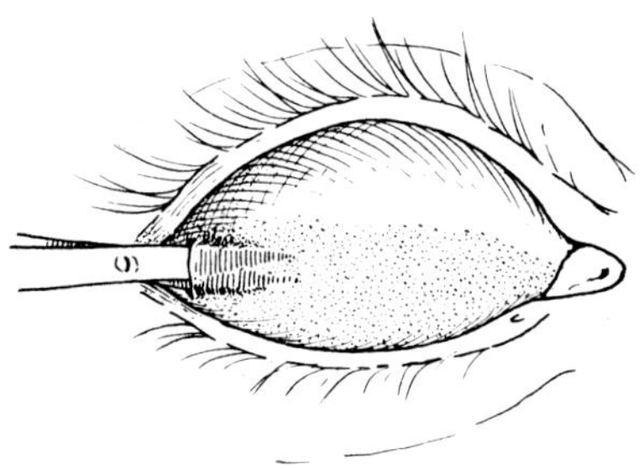

FIG. 7. A scissors is introduced and the conjunctiva is adequately freed.

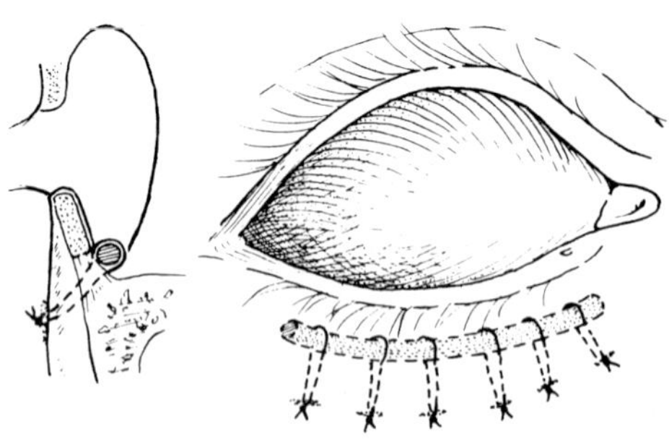

FIG. 8. Sutures of 4-0 silk are looped over a silicone rod, brought out above the orbital rim and tied over cotton bolsters.

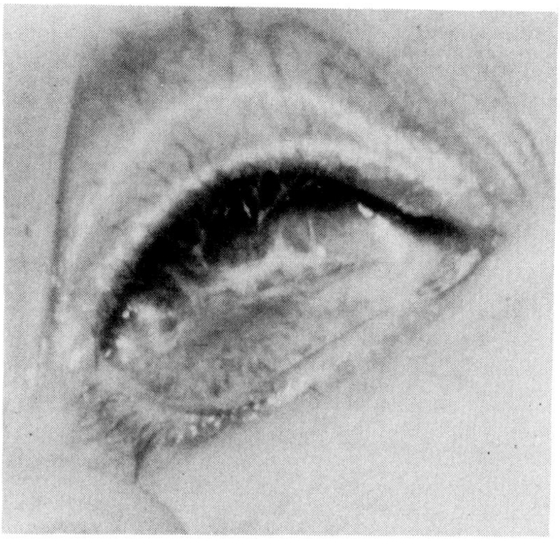

FIG. 9. Absence of lower fornix due to excessive scarring and an inadequate amount of conjunctiva.

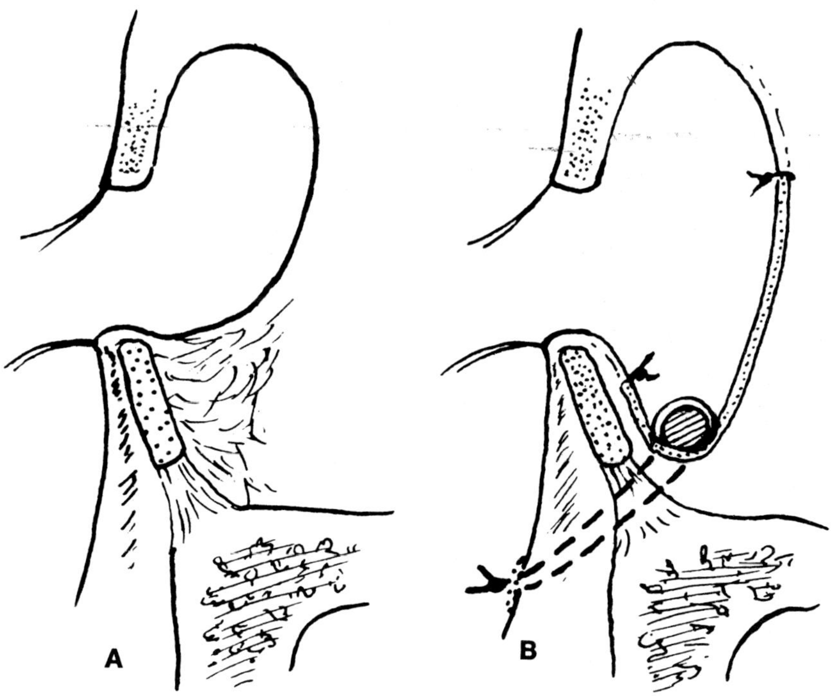

FIG. 10. (A) Severely scarred lower fornix. (B) Re-formation of lower fornix with oral mucous membrane graft. The 4-0 silk sutures are looped around a silicone rod, brought through the skin above the orbital rim and tied over cotton bolsters.

Ectropion

Ectropion may be caused by relaxation of the supporting tissues due to weakness resulting from tissue degeneration or inadequate motor nerve supply. It often begins with ectropion of the lower punctum and epiphora. This may be aggravated by the continuous wiping downward with a handkerchief; this mechanism may aid in the production of a complete ectropion. At the same time the lower lid may sag downward. This leads to poor appearance, epiphora and conjunctival inflammation. With it there may be an increasing difficulty in wearing an artificial eye.

Many modifications of the Kuhnt-Sezymanowski operation have been used to correct ectropion successfully. We prefer correction of ectropion by excising a full-thickness section or wedge, as required, from the lower lid. If necessary, a spindle-shaped resection can be made below the inferior punctum on the conjunctival side and closed with 6-0 chromic sutures, thus causing the punctum to be turned into the tear lake. In less severe cases a row of cautery punctures will do. The medial canthus may be closed temporarily with three sutures tied over a cotton bolster (Figs. 11 and 12).

Three methods of correction of ectropion will be presented. The first is favored by one author (M.J.R.) and the other two by the other author (C.K.B.).

The first method (M.J.R.) employs a segment or wedge resection of the lower lid, usually placed in the lateral third. The term wedge resection is generally misused, for one frequently makes the sides parallel; the wedge-shaped resection is reserved for more severe ectropion. One makes an incision, then grasps the two parts with forceps, draws them together and thus estimates the amount to be removed. After the resection is completed the muscle-fascia layer is freed from the tarsus 2 to 3 mm, and the skin from the muscle-fascia layer the same amount. This aids in the later placement of sutures. Two 7-0 silk sutures are inserted in the lid margin, one anteriorly and one posteriorly. The assistant pulls on each suture, bringing the margin together. The third suture is placed at the gray line, each bite being a little farther back to counteract notch formation. The three sutures are held up by the assistant, thus bringing the tarsal surfaces together. The tarsus is sutured with 6-0 Mersiline or Supramid, passing only halfway through the tissue. They are tied with three knots and the tips' "whiskers" are gently touched with a small cautery to remove them. The muscle-fascia layer is closed with 6-0 chromic gut; usually four sutures are adequate. The margin sutures are tied and the ends left long. The skin is closed with 6-0 Mersiline or silk. The three lid margin sutures

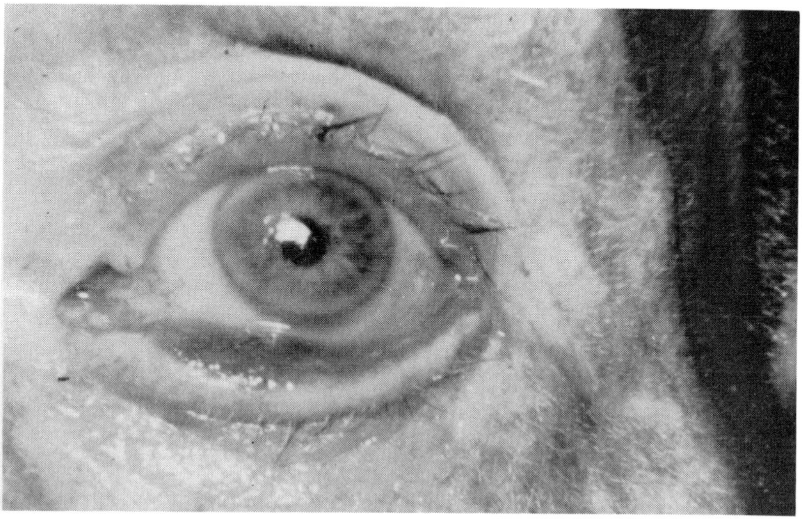

FIG. 11. Relaxation ectropion in an elderly man.

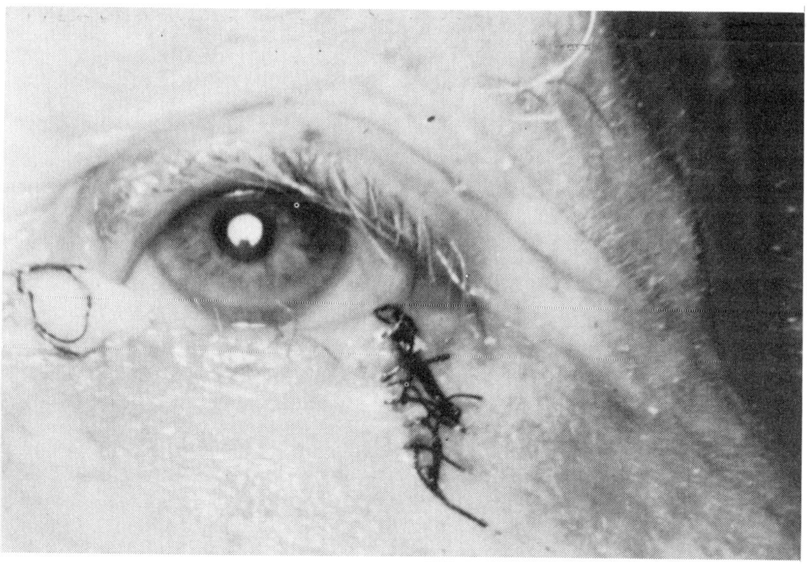

FIG. 12. Postoperative appearance after one week. A wedge-type resection of the lid, spindle resection below the lower punctum and temporary closure of the canthus were performed.

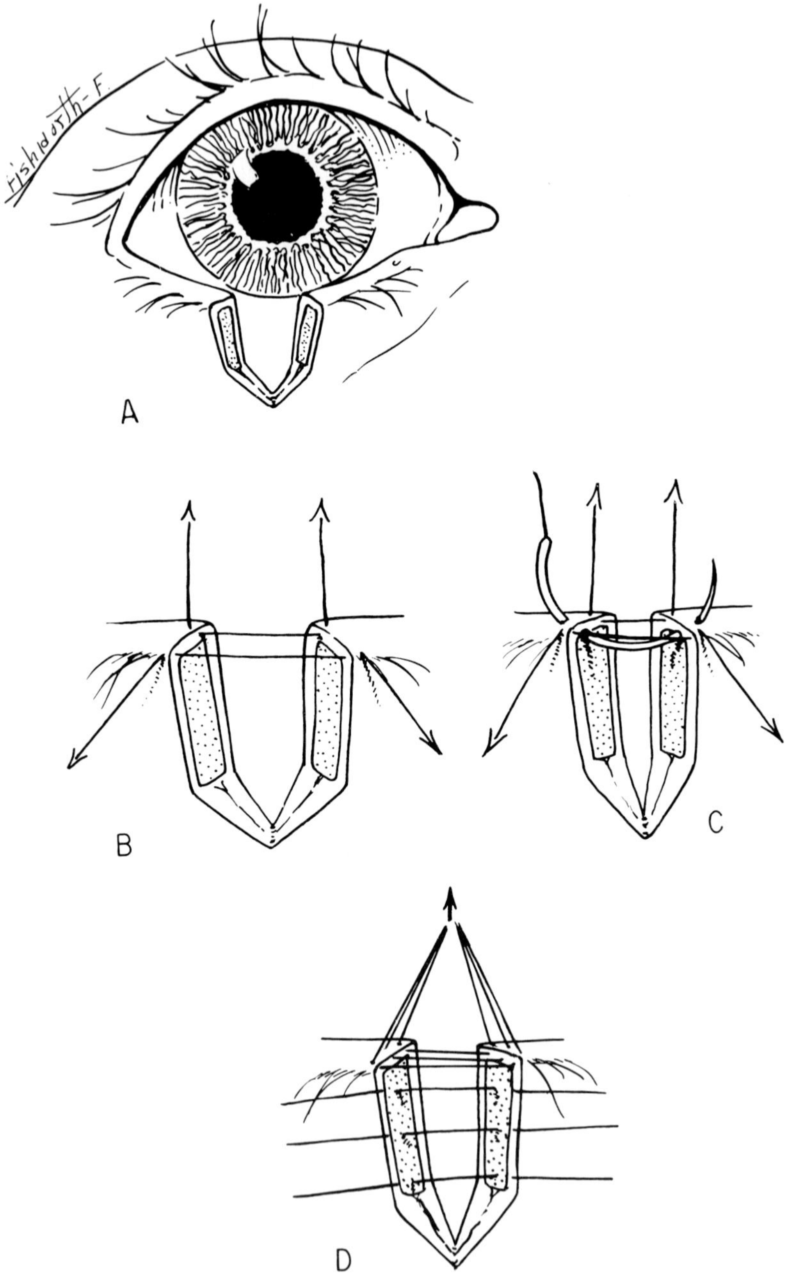
A
B
C
D

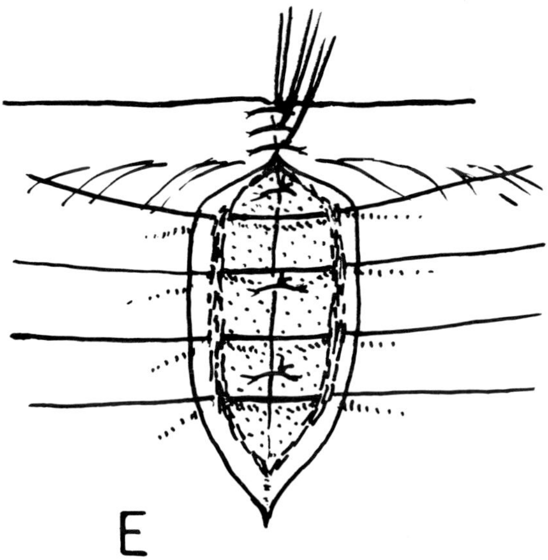

FIG. 13. (A) Excision of required amount of lid. (B and C) Two 7-0 silk sutures are inserted; one is pulled toward the eye and the other away, drawing the wound together; the third margin suture is then inserted. (D) The three margin sutures are held up, bringing the tarsal surfaces together. Usually two 6-0 Mersiline or Supramid sutures are inserted halfway through the tarsal thickness and tied. The "whiskers" are removed with a small cautery. (E) The muscle-fascia layer is closed with four 6-0 chromic gut sutures. (F and G) The skin is closed with 6-0 Mersiline or silk, the three lid margin sutures being incorporated into the top skin suture. The lid has been closed in three layers instead of two.

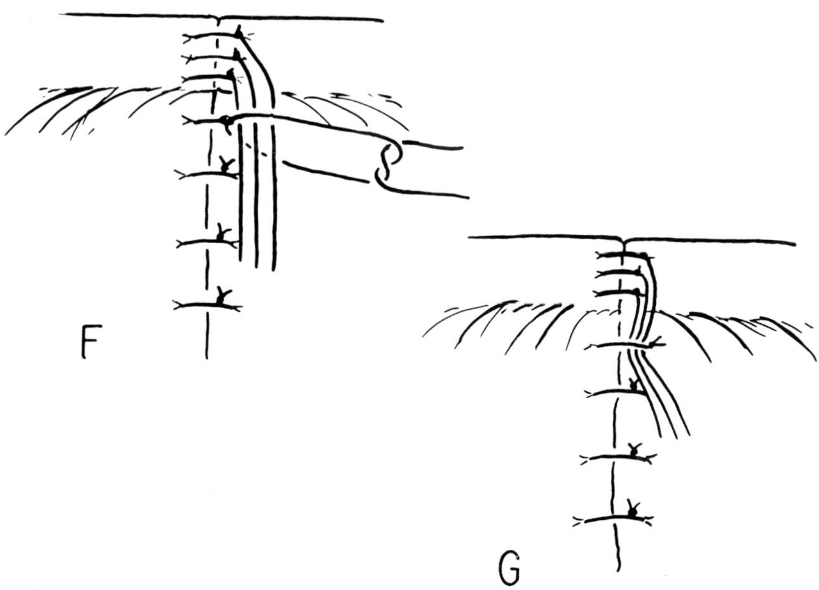

are gathered together and incorporated into the skin suture lying below the lash line. The skin sutures are removed in 6 to 7 days and the lid margin sutures later, 10 to 12 days. This closure is made in three layers instead of two in order to produce a more normal-appearing lid (Fig. 13).

C.K.B. excises the required amount of lid in the lateral third but effects the closure in a slightly different manner. Two 4-0 silk sutures are passed through the skin and muscle and then halfway through the tarsus. Two 6-0 chromic gut sutures are passed only through half the tarsus. These sutures are tied. The skin is closed with 6-0 silk; one 6-0 silk suture is used to close the lid margin. It is left long and taped to the forehead. This is cut short at the first dressing. The skin sutures are removed in 6 to 7 days and the margin sutures in 10 to 12 days (Fig. 14).

C.K.B. has devised an excellent operation for those cases with severe ectropion and loose, degenerated skin. The line of skin incision is outlined with brilliant green (in 95% alcohol), or gentian violet, on the tip of a toothpick. The skin is incised, producing a flap; the amount needed to tighten the lid is removed from the ends at the inverted V-shaped portion. The required excision of lid is carried out, usually toward the lateral half to avoid irritation of the apex of the cornea. The lid margin is closed with three 7-0 silk sutures, tied and left long. The tarsal wound is closed with two 6-0 chromic gut sutures, passed only halfway through the tarsus. The skin is closed with interrupted 6-0 silk sutures. If necessary, skin may be removed in the region of the closure of the tarsal wound. The three lid margin sutures are taped temporarily to the forehead (Fig. 15).

Cicatricial ectropion results from scarring of the skin due to burns; contracting, degenerated or diseased skin; traumatic wounds; or excessive removal of skin when a tumor is excised or a blepharoplasty is performed. One should remember that ectropion associated with deficient skin must be corrected by adding skin, usually in the form of a graft; it is unwise to attempt closure by another procedure without correcting the skin deficiency at the same time. *Deficient skin requires replacement of skin.*

One releases the contracture by making a horizontal incision, carried beyond the commissures when necessary. The skin and muscle are freed adequately and the scar tissue is removed meticulously. This is carried out until the lid comes up with ease. *All* bleeding is stopped with electrocoagulation, avoiding gut ligatures. The bed must be dry. Three sutures of 4-0 silk are inserted in the lid margin or passed from the conjunctival surface through the lid margin to be taped to the forehead for approximately a week. This keeps the lid on the stretch, permitting the graft to be seated without wrinkling. The skin from the upper lid or from behind the ear is preferred. The latter may be better when the lower lid skin is thick in appearance; it must be made 20% larger than the bed,

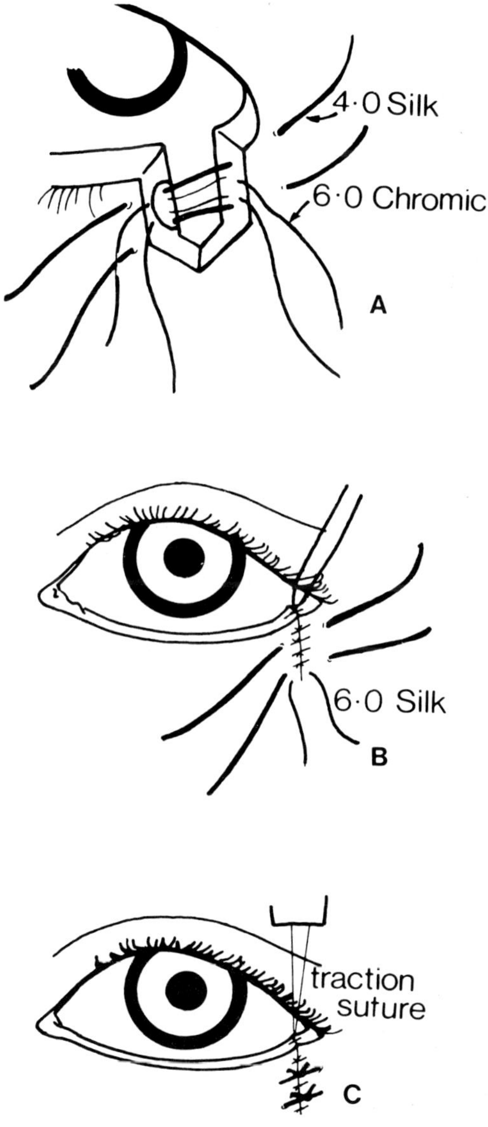

FIG. 14. (A) The required amount of lid has been removed. The wound is closed with two 4-0 silk sutures and two 6-0 chromic sutures. They are passed halfway through the tarsus. (B) The 6-0 chromic gut sutures are tied; the skin and lid margin are closed with 6-0 silk. (C) The 4-0 silk sutures are tied and the margin suture taped to the forehead.

BEYER METHOD

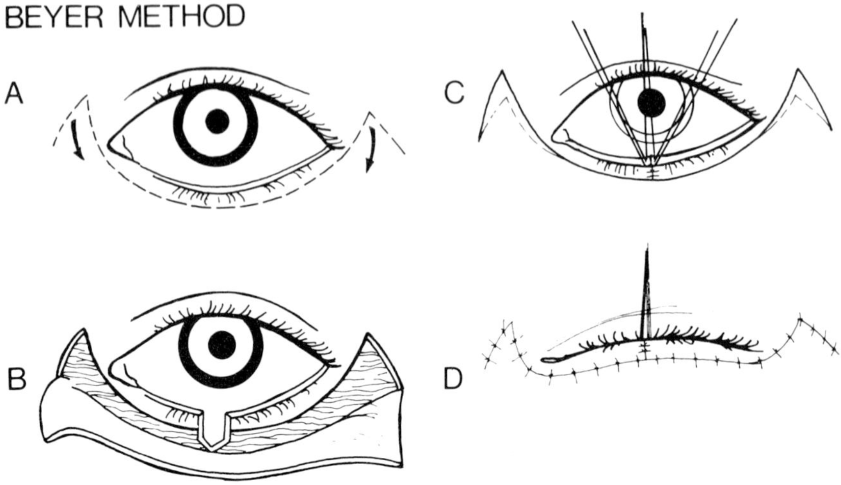

FIG. 15. (A) Skin is marked and incised, producing skin flap. (B) Flap is drawn down and the required amount of tarsus excised, usually toward the lateral half to avoid the corneal apex. (C) Lid margin is closed with three 7-0 silk sutures; tarsus is closed with 6-0 chromic gut. Excess skin is removed at each end. Skin may or may not be removed near the tarsal wound. (D) The skin wound is closed with 6-0 silk; the lid margin sutures, which have been tied, are taped temporarily to the forehead. They are cut short at the first dressing and removed in 10 to 12 days, while the skin sutures are removed in 6 to 7 days.

REPAIR of CICATRICIAL ECTROPION

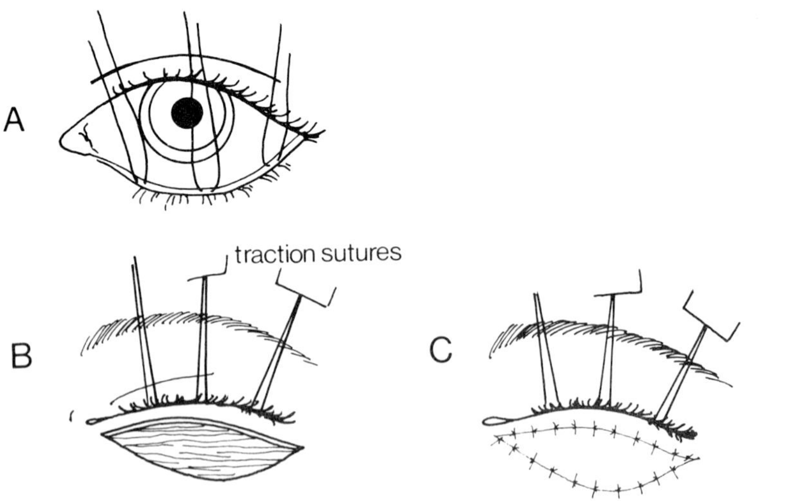

FIG. 16. (A) Three mattress, 4-0 silk sutures are inserted, to be used as traction sutures putting the lid on a stretch. (B) Scar is excised; bed is made *dry*; size of graft needed is determined and a pattern formed. (C) Graft is sutured to bed and proper dressing applied.

whereas upper lid skin can be made the same size. A piece of aluminum foil or the aluminum used to encase the suture material may be shaped and used as a pattern. It is placed over the donor site and outlined with dots from a toothpick dipped in brilliant green in 95% alcohol or gentian violet. One estimates the 20% enlargement of the retroauricular graft. The graft is removed. One must remove only skin, not deeper tissues. The retroauricular graft may be turned over the index finger, raw surface out, and the excess tissue carefully removed with a small scissors. The graft is placed on the *dry* bed and sutured into position with 6-0 silk or Mersiline. A small amount of ointment may be placed on the sutures. Telfa may be placed over the graft. A dental cotton roll usually gives the right amount of pressure over the graft. When this is in place two eye pads are applied and taped in position, producing a reasonable amount of pressure. Wrap-around head dressings are not recommended; if they are used they must not be too tight. The skin sutures are removed, usually half in a week and the remainder two to three days later. A dressing must be maintained until the graft has acquired good contact with the bed and skin margins. The period of dressing will vary; one should avoid leaving the lid exposed and moving until the life of the graft is secure. We emphasize that the bleeding must be controlled, for a hematoma under the graft may lead to a failure. The surgeon, or a trained assistant, should apply the dressing since this is a vital part of the operation. At first the lid will be too high, but healing and scar contracture will draw it down. One seldom needs intermarginal adhesions, especially if the scar has been carefully excised, the lid put on some stretch and the graft placed on a dry bed (Fig. 16).

Bibliography

Beard, C. and Quickert, M. H.: Anatomy of the Orbit. Birmingham, Ala.:Aesculapius Publishing Co., 1969.

Beyer, C. K. and Carrol, J. M.: Moderately severe cicatricial entropion. Arch. Ophthal., 74:327, Aug. 1972.

Butler, J. B. V.: A simple operation for entropion. Arch. Ophthal. 40:665, Dec. 1948.

Cole, J. G.: Amer. Academy Ophthal. & Otolaryng. Teaching Course, Dallas, Texas, 1974.

Guibor, P. and Gougelmann, H. P. (eds.): Problems and Treatment of Contracted Sockets, Exenterated Orbits and Alkali Burns. Miami:Symposia Specialists, 1973.

Jones, L. T., Reeh, M. J. and Wirtschafter, J. D.: Ophthalmic Anatomy (Amer. Acad. Ophthal. & Otolaryng. Manual). Rochester, Minn.:Custom Printing, Inc., 1970.

Jones, L. T., Reeh, M. J. and Wobig, J. L.: Senile entropion. Amer. J. Ophthal., 74:327, Aug. 1972.

Reeh, M. J.: Canthus reconstruction. Ophthal. Surg., vol 1, May-June 1970.

Smith, B. and Cherubini, T.D.: Oculoplastic Surgery. St. Louis:C. V. Mosby Co., 1970.

II. Orbits

- Fractures
- Orbital Tumors
- Congenital Deformities

Prosthetic Shaping and Orbital Displacement to Camouflage Enophthalmos and Bony Deformities

Walter G. Spohn, Ps.D.

A New Team Approach

Much has been said regarding enophthalmos. These deformities were accepted 30 years ago when the ophthalmic plastic surgeon was virtually unknown. Anaplastology* was in its infancy in this country and there was virtually no communication between ocularists. The ophthalmologist would enucleate the eye and dismiss the patient forever, considering that with the removal of the eye, his responsibility was concluded.

Traumatic cases present difficult challenges. Therefore, it is imperative that only custom fitting procedures be employed.

About ten years ago at one of our annual meetings in New York, I presented a paper on "Superior Sulcus Deformities and Ptosis," describing the use of the sulcus crutch. I also suggested the use of a shallow groove near the lower edge of the prosthesis, following the natural curvature of the normal lower eyelid.

We have followed that procedure but found that in many cases the prostheses were too heavy and the patients would develop ptosis in their lower eyelids. This led us to making the eyes hollow (if they were large) to reduce their weight. This procedure was found to be satisfactory, but on reexamining these patients after a number of years, we found that quite a large percentage still developed a sagging lower eyelid.

After World War II and the Korean War, a new breed of ophthalmologists, plastic surgeons and ocularists came to the foreground. They were not satisfied with the accomplishments of the past and endeavored to gain better cosmetic results.

---

*A combination of ocularist and anatomical prosthetist. Presently, this subject is taught at Stanford University and Foothill College, Los Altos Hills, Calif.

Walter G. Spohn, Ps.D., Director, Anaplastology-Ocularist Unit, Department of Surgery, Stanford University School of Medicine, Stanford, Calif.

In our profession as anaplastologists we became closely associated with plastic surgeons during the Vietnam conflict. This relationship developed into a close cooperative venture, including ophthalmologists, plastic surgeons, ENT surgeons and neurosurgeons. Today, we at Stanford work together as a team, enjoying harmonious relationships which result in optimum care for our patients.

Etiology

Following an enucleation and fitting of the prosthesis, one frequently encounters enophthalmos associated with superior sulcus exaggeration. Stone, De Voe and Pheiffer, quoted by Iverson et al [1], mention four possible causes:

1. Malposition of the superior rectus muscle, with its attachments to the levator muscle causing the levator to pull posteriorly rather than superiorly.
2. Loss of volume when the globe is removed.
3. Atrophy of orbital fat.
4. Depression of the floor of the orbit, due to an unrecognized fracture in the orbital floor in the rare case.

Most ocularists feel that a loss of volume in the orbit will result in enophthalmos as well as depression of the upper lid sulcus. These are cosmetic deformities which cannot always be corrected satisfactorily with the prosthesis alone.

Treatment

To correct the volume deficiency and the inferior displacement, depending upon the size of the orbital cavity, the possibility exists that a properly fitting prosthesis may be made, provided the prosthesis is hollow; but the best approach is the team approach – ophthalmologist and ocularist or anaplastologist working as a team:

1. The ocularist makes a prosthesis the size he thinks the patient should have *after surgery*. This prosthesis will look too small but the ophthalmoplastic surgeon will be able to determine the volume that is needed.
2. The method of correction using Silastic RTV was described by Iverson [1].
3. The ocularist or anaplastologist should scrub for surgery with the ophthalmoplastic surgeon and/or ophthalmologist. He should mix the proper RTV and have it in readiness to be placed in position.

4. Prior to mixing the RTV, the ocularist should see that the prosthesis is in the orbit. As the surgeon places the RTV into the desired area, he must watch the artificial eye and stop when the palpebral fissure is of comparative spacing to the living eye. After about five minutes the tubing is removed and the periosteal closure is completed.
5. After six weeks the prosthesis is checked and adjustments are made, if necessary.

How To Make the Prosthesis

When a custom-fitting prosthesis is being designed, the patient should be in an upright sitting position, looking forward at a designated object. We start by examining the socket and carve from pink-base plate wax, a Snellen-type conformer with an iris waxed in the center. The stem of the iris button serves as a handle and also helps in aligning the iris to the proper prominence and spacing.

The wax pattern is perforated with a No. 7 wax spatula, making about five holes. This is to permit the alginate to flow through when taking the impression and also to prevent distortion of contour of the socket.

Making the Alginate Impression

Mix 3-4 cc of alginate to the consistency of soft ice cream and place into a 5-cc syringe. Insert the wax form into the socket; hold the stem with the left hand and with the right hand place the syringe into one of the holes in the wax conformer; inject the alginate into the socket slowly until the material flows out of the holes. At the same time, pull gently on the stem and hold this position until the material is set, about one to two minutes. When investing make sure that the alginate side is invested into the bottom flask* with the stem pointing up.

After the bottom half is firm, trim any excess alginate from the top of the wax pattern and then pour the second half. When the stone is set, the flask is separated, the alginate is removed and a wax pattern is made.

Wax Pattern

Wax is softened in hot water and a sheet of vinyl 0.001 inch in thickness is placed over one half of the mold (acting as the separator). The iris button is replaced and the stem is pushed through the vinyl sheeting into the space left previously. The softened wax, *not melted wax,* is now pressed into the mold cavity, permitting some excess. Another sheet of

*We prefer Hue-Lon Flask made by Caulk, 5 cm × 22 mm each half.

vinyl is placed on top and the flask is closed tightly in a cold press for a few minutes. The flask is opened and the wax form removed.

This is the exact replica of the socket in wax, with the iris in the center, but not necessarily in its proper position.

The Final Impression

The wax pattern is placed into the patient's socket, and the ocularist must now use his skill to properly shape the wax form by adding or eliminating at various areas in order to gain the optimum fit from which he will make the final mold for the eye prosthesis.

Making the Mold

When investing the final wax pattern, make sure that the stem is pointing down and put it into the dental stone until the bottom of the flask is felt. (The stem should have tin foil wrapped around it.) This is necessary for easy removal later. Should one have strong undercuts, then it will be necessary to make a three-piece mold. This can readily be accomplished by the use of RTV Silastic (Fig. 1). Use this as the center portion of the mold; it will prevent the prosthesis form being damaged and it will take the guesswork out of the final finishing of the prosthesis.

Removing the Prosthesis

To remove the prosthesis simply take the shaft of an old or broken dental bur, knock the stem from the back of the flask, and the prosthesis will come out smoothly.

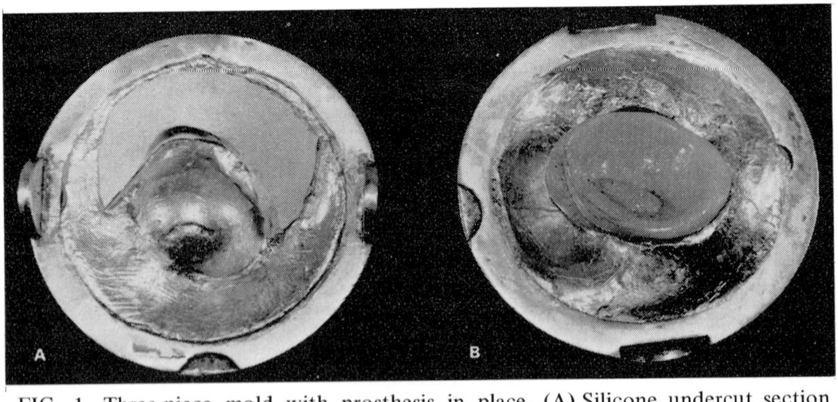

FIG. 1. Three-piece mold with prosthesis in place. (A) Silicone undercut section in place. (B) Prosthesis in second half of mold.

How to Make a Hollow Prosthesis

The wax model is invested, as mentioned above, leaving approximately 3-4 mm exposed so that the remaining exposed area will be in the second half of the flask. When the cavity is filled flush, a sheet of vinyl is placed over the material. The second half is now filled and the two halves are placed in a press and cured as usual. In separating the flask one will find that the eye is in one piece. The prosthesis is polished and tried in the patient's socket prior to adding the simulated blood vessels, etc.

Next the prosthesis is separated where the vinyl sheeting separates the lower part of the prosthesis (where the two halves of the flask meet) (Fig. 2). Both halves are hollowed out to the desired thickness, making sure to leave at least a 2-mm margin where the two halves meet. A thin coating of monopoly syrup or chloropoly solution is painted on the edges of both halves, which are then pressed together in the flask for a few minutes (Fig. 3).

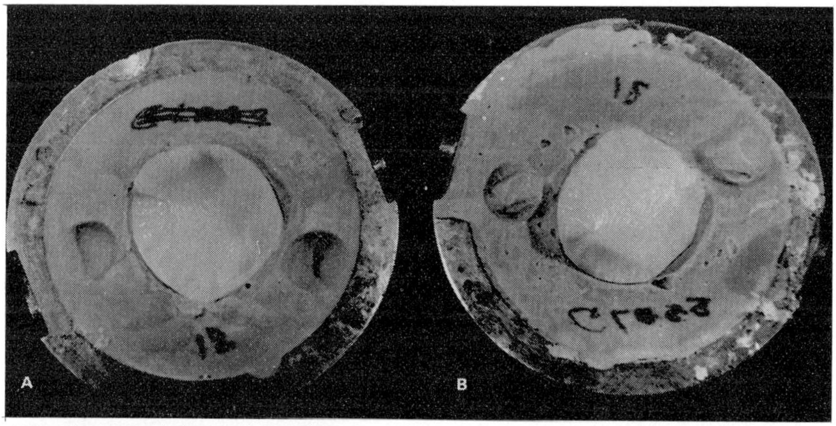

FIG. 2. Both halves of prosthesis in flask after separation and prior to elimination of excess inner material.

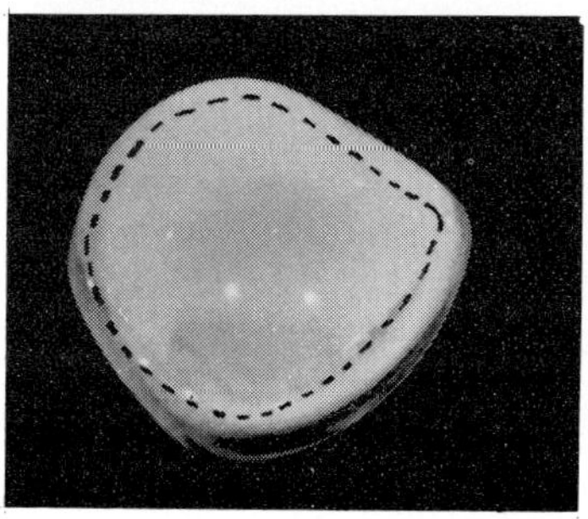

FIG. 3. Back side of prosthesis after the prosthesis has been hollowed out and the two halves have been glued together with chloropoly solution. (Dotted line indicates area that has been hollowed out.)

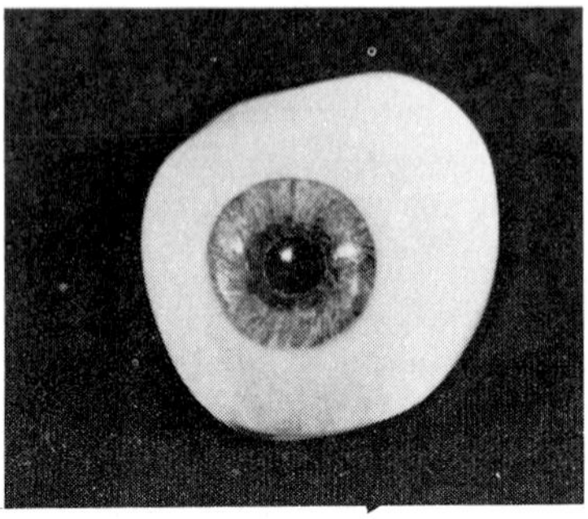

FIG. 4. Front of prosthesis ready to have veining and overlaying pigments applied.

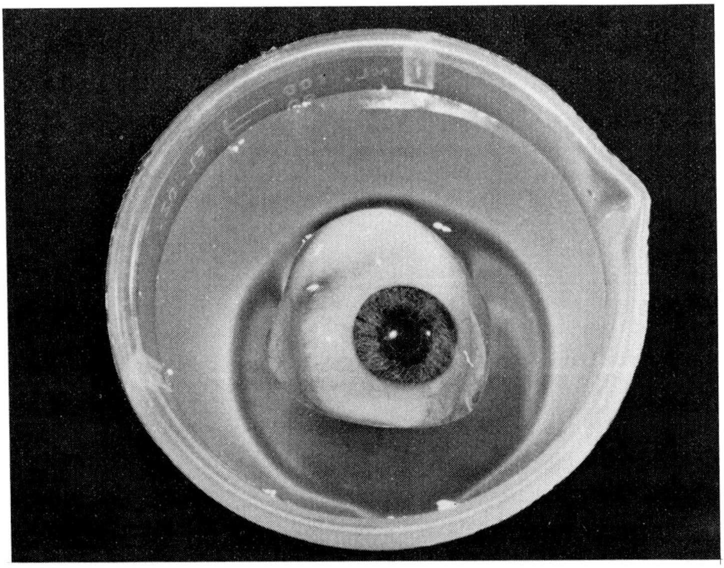

FIG. 5. Completed hollow prosthesis swimming on top of water in a beaker.

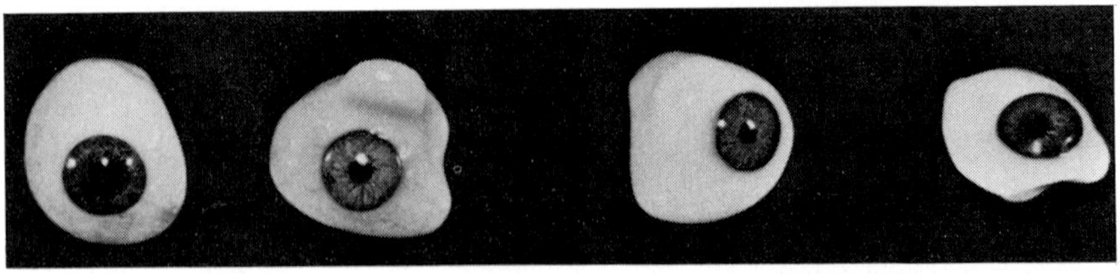

FIG. 6. Various sizes of hollowed-out prostheses.

The prosthesis is now veined and the overlaying pigments are put in place (Fig. 4). The conjunctiva is processed over the entire prosthesis in the usual manner (first trial pack), but in curing, make sure that the iris part is downward during the curing time. Finish the eye as usual, and you will have a prosthesis so light that it will float on water (Fig. 5).

Various types of hollow lightweight prostheses are shown in Figure 6.

Summary

To correct orbital displacements, and to camouflage enophthalmos and bony deformities, various techniques have been tried. Some fine temporary results have been attained, but very little of lasting endurance has been accomplished in the past by the ocularist alone.

Surgically, glass and silicone beads have been used. The glass beads migrated and moved about, but the silicone beads embedded themselves in bony areas.

The team effort of ophthalmoplastic surgeons and anaplastologists has brought about a change for the better by using RTV Silastic. Great progress has been made by using a combination of RTV and a fascia lata sling, as described by Iverson, Vistnes and Spohn [2].

References

1. Iverson, R. E., Vistnes, L. M. and Siegel, R. J.: Correction of enophthalmos and in the anophthalmic orbit. Plast. Reconstr. Surg. 51:545, 1973.
2. Iverson, R. E., Vistnes, L. M. and Spohn, W.: Repairing superior lid sulcus depression. Today's Ocularist, 1:4, 1973.

Anophthalmic Enophthalmos

Paul T. Gavaris, M.D.

History

The problem of enophthalmos developing in the enucleated orbit has been challenging physicians since the procedure was introduced by Cleobury [1] in 1826. It remained for Mules in 1885 to use a glass sphere as an implant in the eviscerated eye and then two years later for Frost and Lang to insert one into Tenon's capsule. These pioneers, together with the introduction by Snellen of the "reform eye," made the first significant contributions toward preventing this iatrogenic scar. By utilizing modern technological advances in material, further major achievements were made in the last 25 years by inventive surgeons and skilled ocularists.

Causes

The probable causes of enophthalmos include the following:

1. Insufficient volume replacement, the most common and the most significant cause [2, 3]. The volume of an eye is 6.5 cc; that of the orbit is 31 cc. Thus 20% of volume is lost by enucleation alone (Figs. 1-3).
2. Contracture and scarring of fascia and muscle, the amount of which depends on the degree of hemorrhage, edema or trauma sustained by the tissue.
3. Neurotropic atrophy of muscle and fat, which is analogous to other paralytic syndromes.
4. Exaggeration of enophthalmos – noted when an associated rim, floor or trimalar fracture has not been adequately reduced [4].

The opinions or assertions contained herein are those of the author and are not to be construed as official or reflecting the view of the Navy Department of the naval service at large.

Paul T. Gavaris, M.D., Ophthalmologist, National Naval Medical Center, Bethesda, Md.

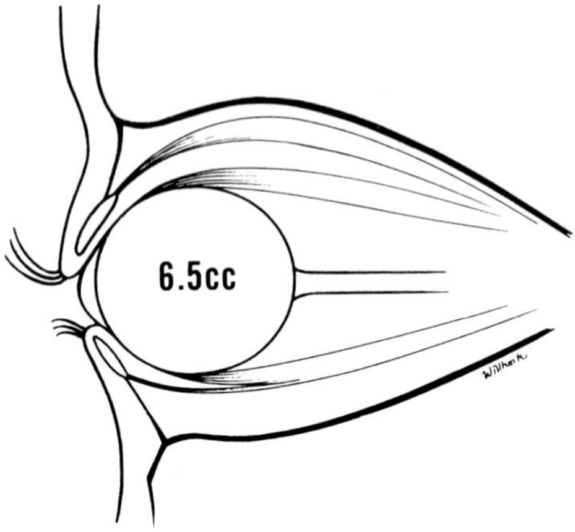

FIG. 1. Normal orbit showing relative globe-orbit volume relationship. Note natural arching of levator and anterior position of globe.

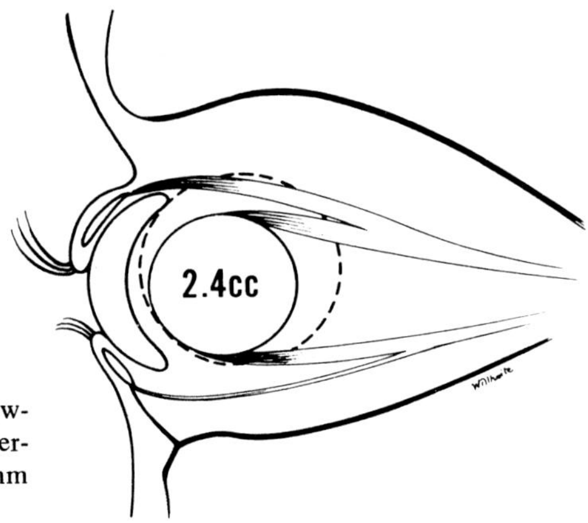

FIG. 2. Enucleated orbit showing loss of volume and moderate sulcus with a 16-mm implant.

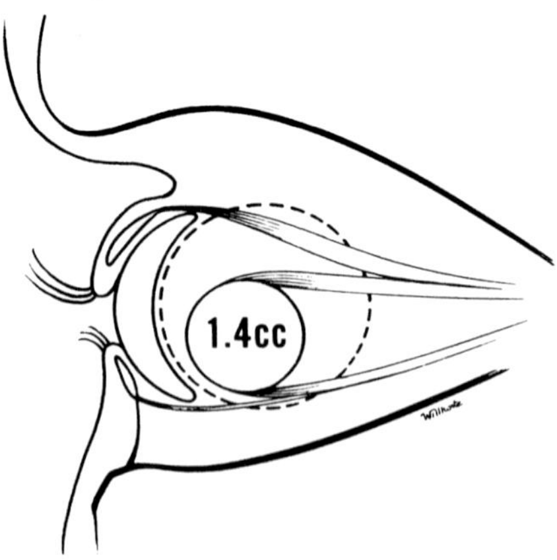

FIG. 3. Enucleated orbit with a 14-mm implant showing severe sulcus, volume loss and tissue realignment.

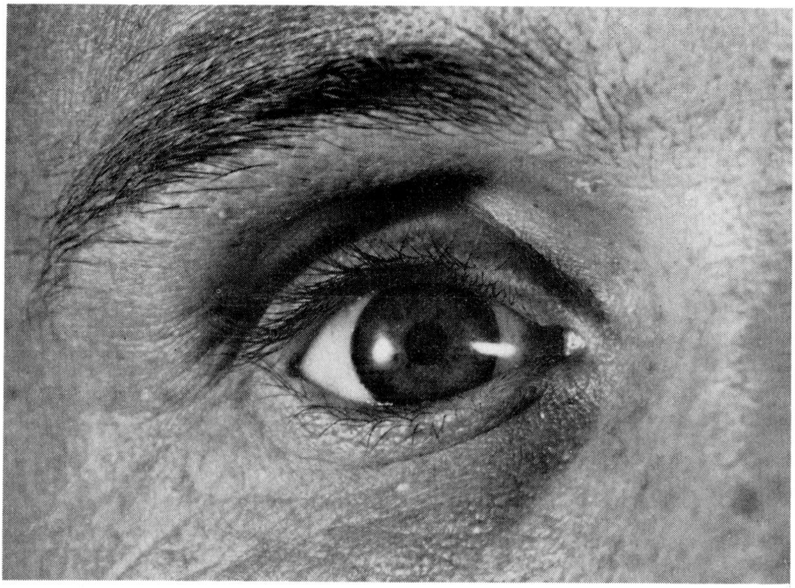

FIG. 4. A 28-year-old man with severe enophthalmos two years after implant extruded.

5. Alteration of the levator-superior rectus relationship, which occurs with loss of the globe or use of an implant less than 16 mm in diameter. The pull of the levator has changed from vertical to a posterior direction, consequently reducing the lid fold, increasing the sulcus and accentuating the enophthalmic appearance. (Compare Figs. 1 and 3.)

In my opinion, the superior sulcus syndrome should not be viewed as a separate entity apart from enophthalmos. To illustrate this point, one can observe the elimination of the sulcus by merely pushing on the lower lid of an enophthalmic orbit (Figs. 4 and 5). This suggests that enophthalmos and superior lid sulcus are one and the same, ie, a result of volume loss. Previous modes of treatment with banana-shaped synthetics [5] and fascial, dermal or fat grafts, though very ingenious, are at best poor attempts to camouflage. The goal of treatment should be the restoration of the orbital contents to its original volume.

Treatment

When an orbital fracture is contributing to enophthalmos, it should be corrected first. Using a subciliary incision and creating a skin-muscle flap, a pure "blowout" may be reduced by the method described by Smith and

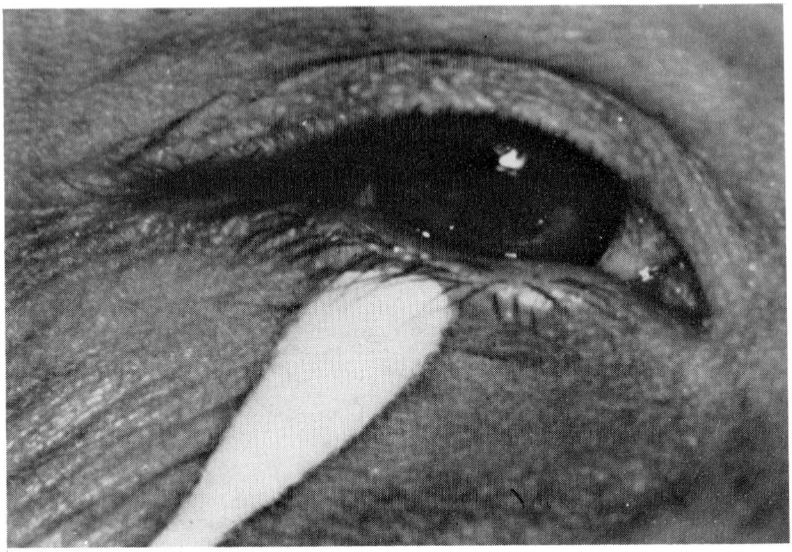

FIG. 5. Same patient showing marked improvement of sulcus merely by pushing in on lower lid.

Putterman [6]. Segmental telescoping of the rim or a displacement of the malar prominence requires open reduction and wiring of the segments as soon as possible. If the trauma is old, reconstruction of any defects can be accomplished with either bone autografts, Cranioplast (shaped during its exothermic polymerizing stage) or preformed silicone rubber forms.

The presence of an implant within the muscle cone is necessary for optimum results. For example, an 18-mm implant (3.2 cc) restores almost half of the globe volume, restores the natural arching of the levator and reduces the socket depth – allowing for a thinner prosthesis and better motility. A late or secondary implant of at least 16-18 mm can be inserted via the direct conjunctival or the lateral brow approach described by Iliff [7]. The use of glass or silicone beads in lieu of a sphere greatly reduces the potential for motility. An integrated implant or one to which the recti can be sutured may reduce the incidence of migration and extrusion.

A residual enophthalmos, ie, 2 mm or more, may be managed by several imaginative procedures. These include the use of bone or fascial grafts [8]; Teflon, Silastic or Supramid wedges [3]; Teflon "dog sled" orbital floor implant [9]; glass beads at the orbital apex [10]; inflatable subperiosteal implants [11] or RTV Medical Silastic 382 implantation reported initially by Hill [12] in 1965 and more recently by Iverson [13].

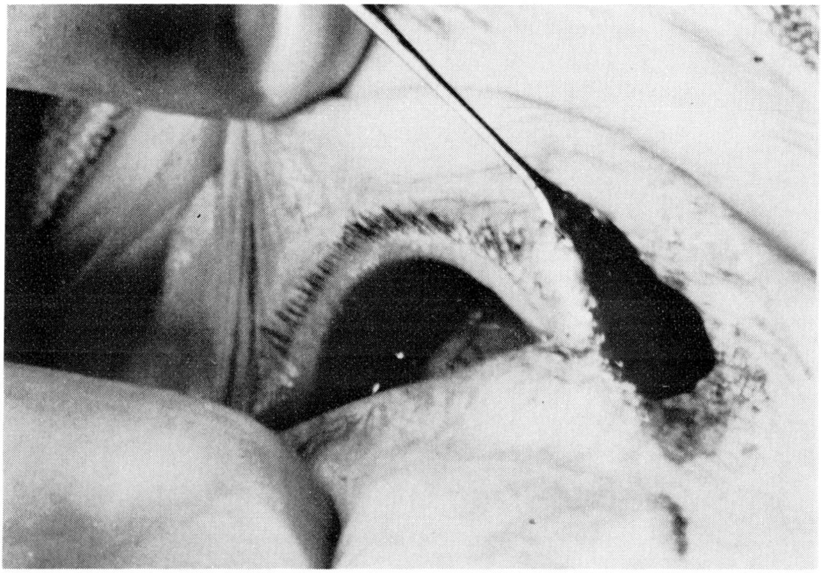

FIG. 6. An anophthalmic orbit showing dissection into subperiosteal space via lateral canthal incision.

In the author's opinion, the use of Silastic 382 offers several advantages and will be described in detail.

Pre- and postoperative socket hygiene, facial scrubs, topical and systemic antibiotics are prescribed routinely. After intubation and a meticulous prep, a 15-mm incision is made along the lateral rim, 5 mm from the canthus, through skin, muscle and periosteum. With a periosteal elevator the arcus marginalis is elevated above and below the tendon insertion. The dissection is carried posteriorly along the lateral, superior and inferior walls, taking care not to perforate the periorbita (Fig. 6). A half-inch gauze tape premoistened in 1:100,000 epinephrine solution is gently packed into this subperiosteal cavity and retained for five minutes. Each 12-gauge intravenous cannula or IV tubing with syringe adapters is directed into the superolateral and inferolateral pockets. The periosteum is sutured on both sides of each tube with Dexon or Tevdek sutures (Fig. 7). The stannous octoate catalyst and monomer are sterilized separately by the method of Hill [12]. A test sample is prepared using enough catalyst for a setting time of eight to ten minutes. A large corneal scleral shell is retained firmly in the socket during, and for ten minutes after, implantation. This step prevents the polymer from dissecting anteriorly

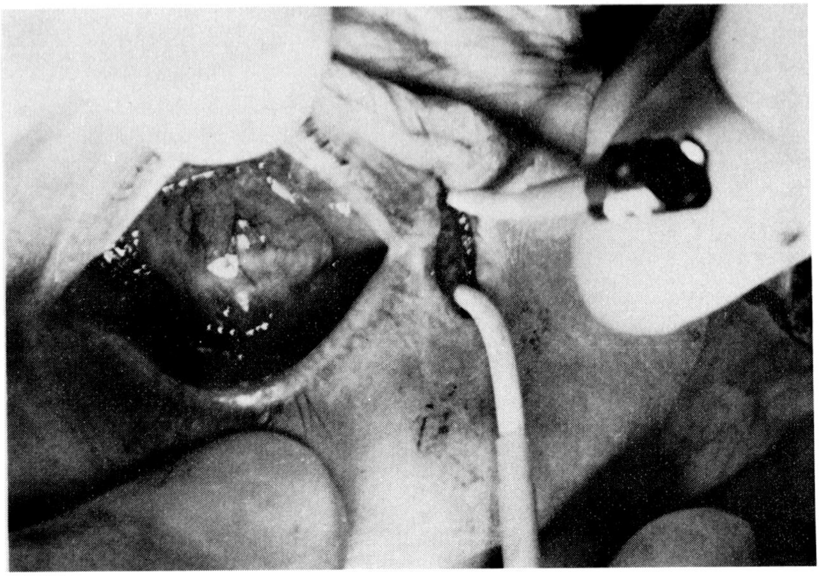

FIG. 7. Both cannulas are secured into the upper and lower pockets prior to implantation of RTV Silastic.

and reducing the fornices. Using two wide-base 10-cc disposable syringes, an equal amount of polymer is squeezed through each syringe until the enophthalmos is reduced completely. An additional 0.5 cc is implanted to compensate for the concurrent edema. The tubing is removed slowly as the Silastic begins to set; any excess is excised with a scalpel or scissors. The periosteum and skin are closed separately with nonreactive synthetic sutures (Fig. 8). A moderate pressure dressing is applied and changed daily for three to four days to retard edema. A new prosthesis can be fashioned in four to six weeks.

Discussion

The advantages of RTV Silastic 382 within the subperiosteal spaces are several (Figs. 9 and 10):

1. Significant volume is readily available.
2. It will not disturb the muscle cone or implant.
3. It squeezes orbital contents outwardly, thus augmenting motility.
4. Silastic will not migrate as do beads.
5. It is essentially nonreactive and can readily be removed completely if necessary.

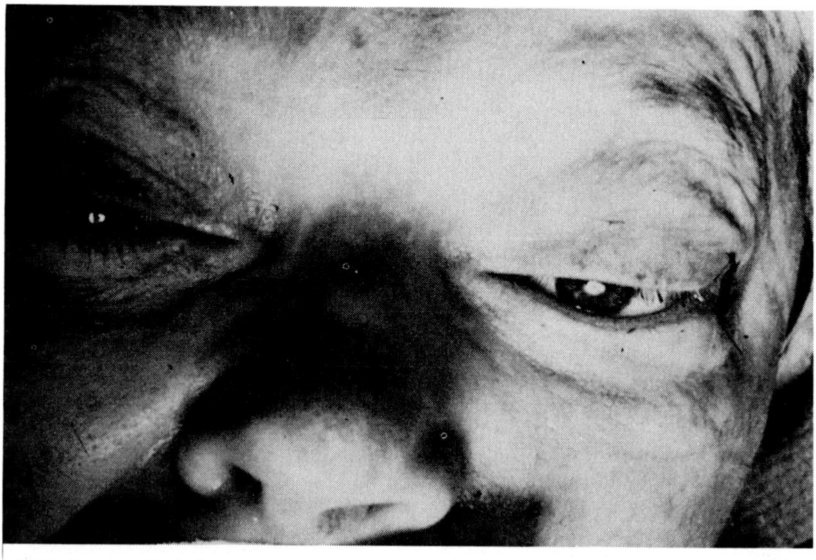

FIG. 8. At end of the procedure the enophthalmos has been completely reduced.

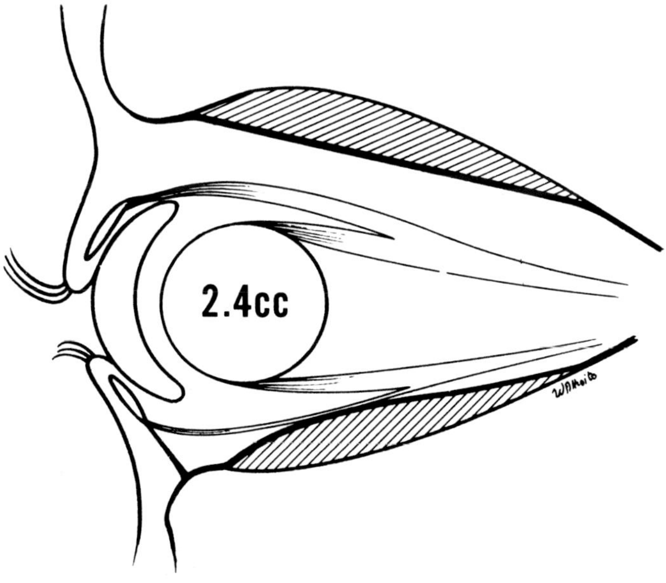

FIG. 9. Schematic orbit with RTV Silastic 382 in the superior and inferior pockets. Note lack of disturbance to muscle cone and implant.

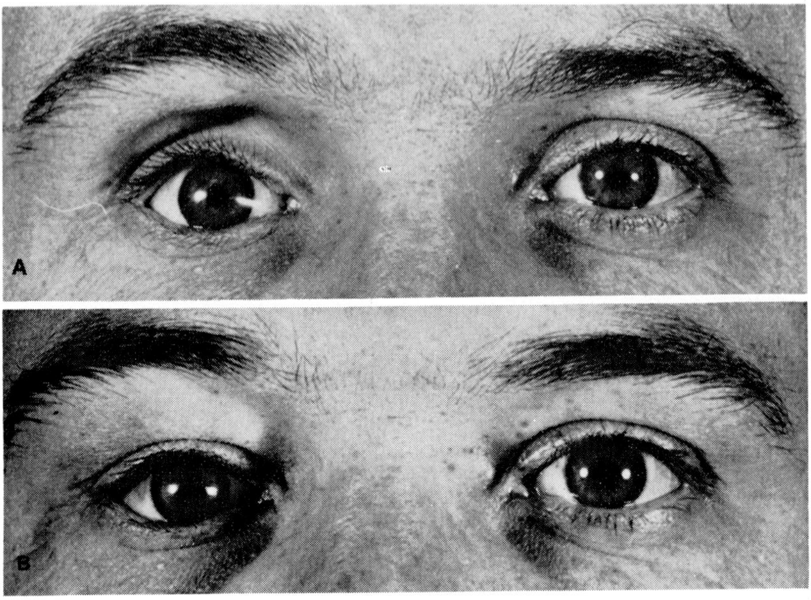

FIG. 10. (A) Preoperatively – a 28-year-old man with 7 mm enophthalmos and marked superior sulcus; (B) Postoperatively – complete improvement after 2.8 cc of Silastic polymer implantation.

Summary

The various aspects of anophthalmic enophthalmos are discussed. The cause of enophthalmos is essentially insufficient volume replacement. The superior sulcus defect should not be thought of as a separate entity, but as synonymous with enophthalmos. A procedure which replaces this volume loss is described in detail and is favored most by this author.

References

1. Cleobury, W.: A review of the different operations performed on the eyes. London:T & G Underwood, 1826, pg. 261.
2. Culler, A. M.: Basic principles of anatomy and physiology of the orbit and relation to implant surgery. Trans. Amer. Acad. Ophthal., 56:17-20, 1972.
3. Sherman, A. E.: The retracted eye socket. Amer. J. Ophthal., 35:89-101, 1952.
4. Hotte, H. H. A.: Orbital Fractures. Assen, Netherlands:Koninklijke Van Gorcum & Co. N.V., 1970.
5. Sugar, H. S. and Forestner, H. I.: Methacrylic resin implants for sunken upper lid following enucleation. Amer. J. Ophthal., 29:993-1000, 1946.
6. Smith, B. and Putterman, A. M.: Fixation of orbital floor implants. Arch. Ophthal., 83:598, 1970.

7. Iliff, C. E.: The extruded implant. Arch. Ophthal., 78:742-744, 1967.
8. Cole, J. G.: Correction of enophthalmos with bone and fascia lata grafts. *In* Smith and Converse (eds.): Plastic and Reconstructive Surgery of the Eye and Adnexa. St. Louis:C. V. Mosby Company, 1967, pp. 450-453.
9. Hneleski, I. S., Jr. and Shannon, G. M.: Orbital floor implant. Amer. J. Ophthal., 76:540-542, October 1973.
10. Guibor, P. and Smith, B.: Orbital glass bead inserter. Trans. Amer. Acad. Ophthal. Otolaryn., 76:259, 1972.
11. Soll, D. B.: Correction of superior lid sulcus with subperiosteal implants. Arch. Ophthal., 85:188-190, 1971.
12. Hill, J. C.: Enophthalmos: Foreign injections. *In* Smith and Converse (eds.): Plastic and Reconstructive Surgery of the Eye and Adnexa. St. Louis:C. V. Mosby Company, 1967, pp. 439-445.
13. Iverson, R. E., Vistnes, L. M. and Siegler, R. J.: Correction of enophthalmos in the anophthalmic orbit. Plast. Reconstr. Surg., 51:5:545, 1973.

Prosthetic Restoration for Exenteration

Frederick R. Lewis

Four types of orbital exenterations are presented to the ocularist for restoration. Most common is the deep socket. The entire contents of the orbit are removed and the remaining bony orbit is skin grafted or tissue is allowed to granulate and cover the area.

Partial removal of the orbital contents results in a shallow socket. It is typical for these sockets to have an opening for drainage of the sinus. This sinus opening is not a problem. The prosthetic replacement can easily be designed to vault the area. A small cotton ball is usually placed in this vault to absorb moisture.

When the eyelids are not involved in the malignancy it is possible to exenterate the orbit and retain the lids. If the lids can be restored to somewhat near their normal positions, they are of real value and can be used to hide and hold the edges of any prosthetic replacement that may follow.

The orbital exenteration process may extend to include ablation of the nose. The nasal area is not so easily covered by a patch or bandage as are the eye and orbit, and the need for prosthetic replacement is increased even though the replacement may be more complex to design and fabricate.

Conditions influencing feasibility of prostheses for orbital exenteration will be discussed later. At this point two facial restorations, the nasal prosthesis and the exenteration prosthesis, are mentioned to sharpen the focus on the particular factors that limit use of the exenteration prosthesis.

It would appear to most observers that the nose, being a prominent feature in the center of the face, would present the greatest problems in cosmetic facial restorations. Yet, in my experience, most patients with

---

Frederick R. Lewis, Ocularist, Beverly Hills, Calif.

ablation of the nose wear a prosthesis. Most patients experiencing orbital exenteration do not wear a prosthesis. Why is this so?

It is true that when the nose is surgically ablated it is extremely difficult to bandage or patch the area without blocking out a good portion of the face. These circumstances encourage patients to wear a prosthetic nose. But this is not the reason for the great disparity in the wearing of the two types of prostheses.

The reason most patients with orbital exenteration do not wear a prosthesis is the lack of symmetry in animation. The eye and eyelids of the restoration do not move like the normal eye and eyelids. The stationary eye and immobile eyelids of the exenteration restoration are made more apparent when, in the same view, the patient's fellow normal eye can be observed moving and functioning freely. It is this rigid, sometimes fixed expression that has caused many orbital exenteration patients to reject a prosthesis. Some practical method of animation of the exenteration prosthesis would be welcomed. Incidence of exenteration of the orbit is relatively infrequent.

Funding is not and probably will not be available for direct research into animation of exenteration prostheses. Any breakthrough will probably come by adapting technology from other fields.

Factors Determining Feasibility of Exenteration Prostheses

There are patients who wear orbital exenteration prostheses with a good degree of success. The following factors determine the feasibility of orbital exenteration restoration:

1. *Age.* Age is a very important consideration. Exenteration prostheses require care that most children are not capable of or responsible to. Wearing an orbital exenteration prosthesis can greatly interfere with the normal activities of children. Growth of the child can cause change in the tissues on which the prosthesis seats, requiring frequent adjustment, renewal and expense. Last, it is extremely difficult to blend the edge of the prosthesis to match the smooth, delicate, wrinkle-free skin of a child. I have not had success in fitting children with exenteration prostheses.

Exenteration restorations can be made for most adults. Older adults have skin with less tone, more folds, blotches and wrinkles. The margins of the orbital restoration can be blended into this irregular type of skin, causing the entire piece to be less apparent, less conspicuous. It is essential that eye glasses be worn in conjunction with the prosthesis to attain the maximum cosmetic value. Many adults ordinarily wear eye glasses and those who do not are usually receptive to using them.

2. *Occupation.* Best candidates for exenteration prostheses are white collar workers or others normally employed indoors away from the elements, grease and grime. Poor candidates are laborers, those employed in heavy industry, auto mechanics, etc.

3. *Motivation.* The patient must want to wear the exenteration prosthesis if it is to be successful. A strong motivation can often make the difference between success and failure in many projects. Patient involvement and an interest in helping himself are essential here.

4. *Extent of ablated area.* If the exenteration process extends out of the orbit into areas of the face where the tissues are very mobile, it may complicate or even prohibit the use of a practical restoration. Motivation and temperament of the patient should be carefully analyzed before proceeding with an expanded case of this nature.

Consultation

Prior to beginning an exenteration prosthesis, consultation with the patient and his family is important. The circumstances surrounding a current case illustrate why.

A 72-year-old woman who resides in Southern California elected to be operated for exenteration in New York. She was operated June this year. The cavity was skin grafted and it has taken well. The right eyebrow has been pulled down and in toward the cavity. This occurs often and does present a problem in design of the prosthetic replacement, but can be coped with. The patient's husband called my office for an appointment while his wife was still convalescing in New York. He showed some anxiety, and the appointment was arranged so that the patient could be seen with her husband present immediately upon their return to California. The consultation was held and all aspects of the proposed restoration were discussed openly and honestly. In response to questions, it was explained that the design of the restoration would aid in its retention to the face, but for the most part the prosthesis would be held in place by adhesives.

Also, it was explained the prosthesis should be removed each night to allow the tissues on which it rests a chance to be exposed to the air. Some patients find the eye socket will tolerate wearing the restoration two or three days at a time. It was suggested that experimentation with a longer wearing time should be attempted only after several months of normal wear.

In response to a third question, they were told the orbit must be well healed, free of crusting and free of sensitive areas before the restoration could be started. It usually takes three to six months for this healing to occur. It is better to delay fabrication of the prosthesis if there is any doubt the area is stable.

I attempted to convey some of the limitations of exenteration prostheses to them, but in this initial visit their state of mind was such that my message was not fully received. Specifics of the prosthesis will be dealt with again in the next visit. At that time the orbit should be healed and future change in the tissues and size of the area should be minimal. If the second consultation with the patient is favorable, impressioning and fabrication of the prosthesis can begin. I believe this patient could be a good candidate for an exenteration prosthesis.

Case Report

A 60-year-old man (Fig. 1) suffered exenteration of the right orbit in 1953 following discovery of a basal cell carcinoma. He was fitted with a prosthesis five months postoperatively and has had periodic replacements since. The patient was gainfully employed as a meatcutter until just recently when he retired on disability due to a condition not related to the exenteration. He has been and still is an active, enthusiastic golfer. The prosthesis shown in Figure 2 is two years old. (This picture was made when he returned to have it "touched up" and have a new piece made.) Wearing eye glasses greatly enhances the cosmetic value of the prosthesis (Fig. 3).

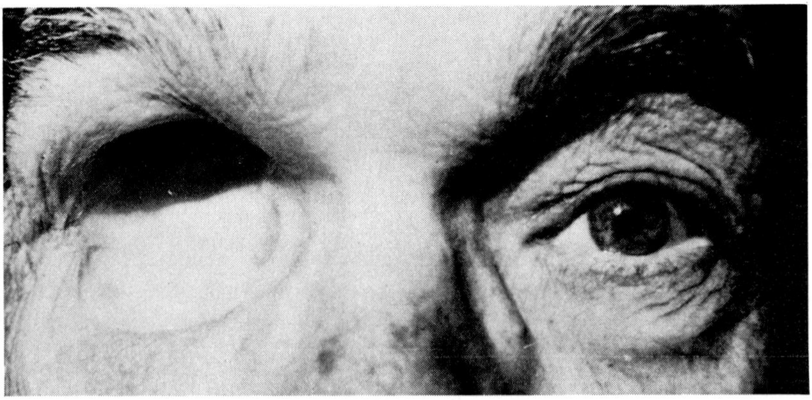

FIGURE 1.

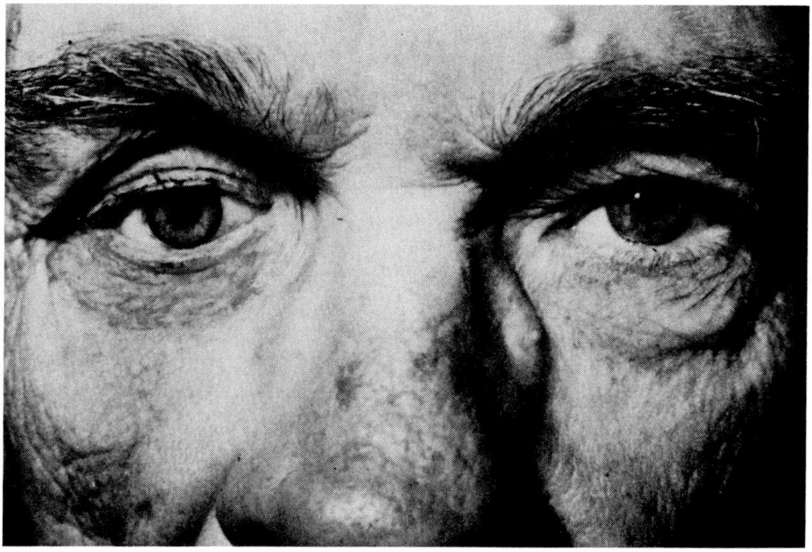

FIGURE 2.

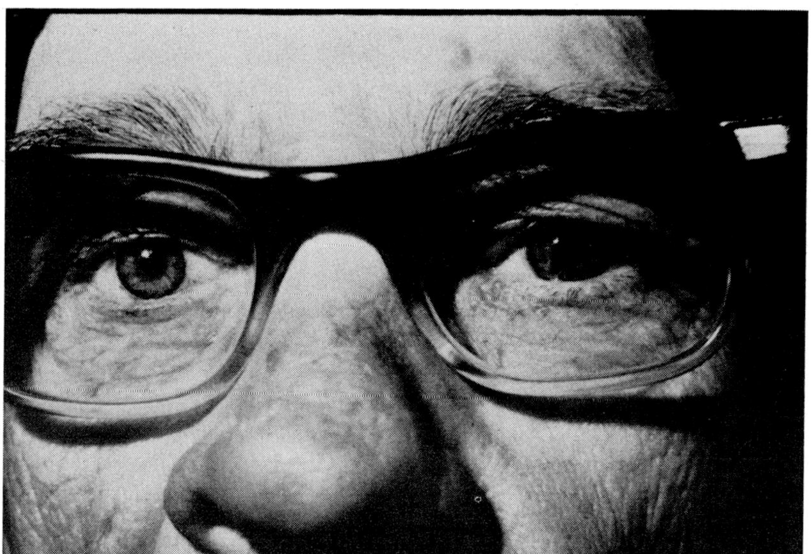

FIGURE 3.

Summary

Types of orbital exenterations presented for restoration by prostheses have been shown. An attempt has been made to focus attention on the primary causes that prohibit more general use of exenteration prostheses. Factors determining feasibility of these prostheses were also discussed. A case history of the successful use of an orbital restoration for 20 years was cited. The challenge to rehabilitate exenteration patients is not a small one. Each attempt toward successful orbital restoration is a step in the right direction.

Atypical Orbital Exenteration

Daniel Silva, M.D.

Exenteration of the orbit is a radical surgical technique that must be reserved for the treatment of malignant diseases starting inside the orbit or coming from or invading the periorbital structures. In a great number of cases a typical exenteration can be performed because of the histologic nature of the tumor, or the limited extent of its growth within the orbital walls. But in many others, where there is extension of the malignancy to the orbital tissues or beyond the orbital periosteum, an atypical exenteration must be performed with oncologic criteria. That means en block resection if possible, or at least concentric removal of diseased tissue from its healthy periphery toward the center of the lesion.

What is a typical orbital exenteration? It is a surgical procedure described almost four centuries ago, whose main technical advance was achieved after Kirby's [1] immediate grafting of the bare cavity with split-thickness skin graft. The technique most suitable to be called typical is the one described by Iliff in 1957 [2], in which the skin incision is made over the orbital rim in a single cut up to the periosteum. This is elevated over as far as the apical stump, which is clamped and neatly cut. The orbital contents are wholly removed and the cavity is packed with gauze. Then the skin graft is sutured to the skin incision, after all hemorrhage has been controlled, and the vascular stump is fulgurated. The cavity is packed with some absorbent material like sea sponge, and a pressure bandage is applied to be removed for dressing after the fifth day, at which time the patient can be released. The healing takes place quickly and a prosthesis can be worn in about five to six weeks (Fig. 1).

This typical orbital exenteration was performed in 61 cases of my described series of 300 consecutive cases of orbital tumors in 1968 [3]. However, a number of changes in the surgical technique had to be made since then, on account of the nature of the tumor, its stage of clinical

Daniel Silva, M.D., Ophthalmology Department, Hospital de Oncologia, Centro Médico Nacional, Mexico City, Mexico.

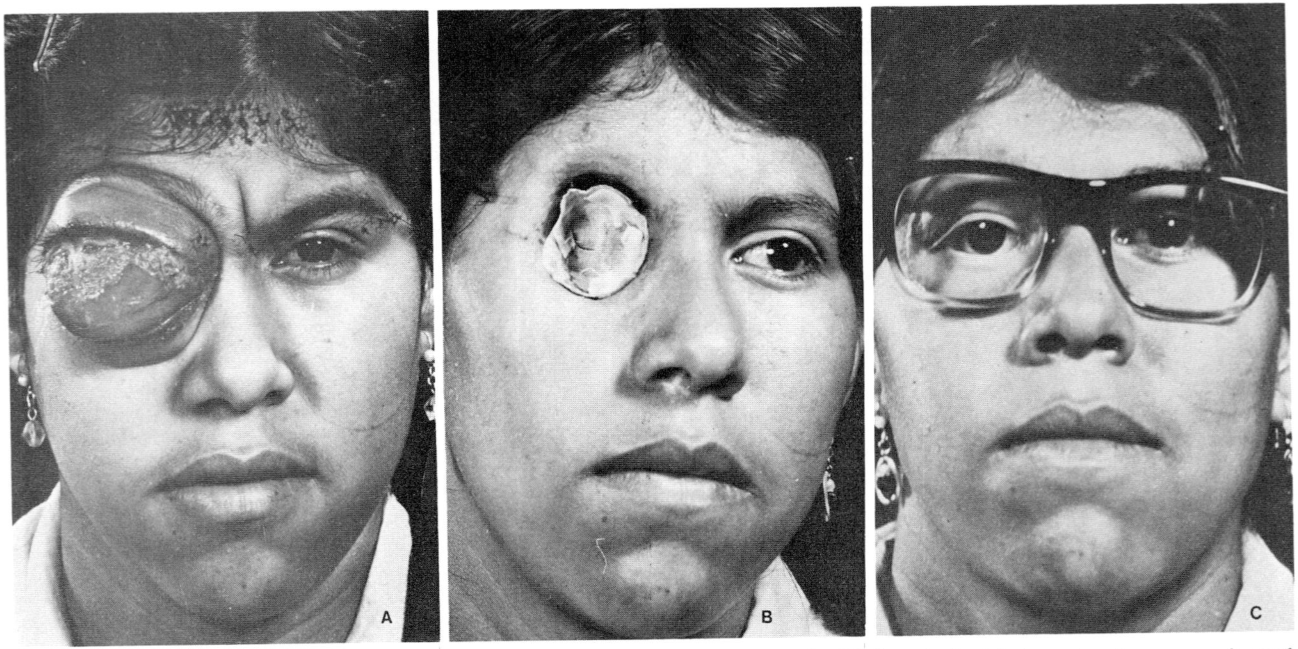

FIG. 1. Typical orbital exenteration. (A) Enormous rabdomyosarcoma of right orbit. (B) A typical orbital exenteration was performed. The cavity was lined with a single organdy layer to avoid damaging the epithelial graft when pressure packing with gauze. (C) Five weeks later a prosthesis mounted on the glasses concealed the surgical blemish.

evolution and the previously used therapy. These modifications can be classified into two main groups: (1) when the purpose was to minimize the surgical injury and to achieve immediate satisfactory cosmesis, and (2) when the goal was to perform a radical excision of the tumor with wide safety margins.

The first group becomes atypical by three main variations:

1. *By omitting the skin grafting,* the orbital cavity being allowed to fill up with granulation tissue. This old technique may give some good cosmetic results, but the healing takes place very slowly and often complications arise: infection, suppurative drainage of some ethmoidal cavities and the most dreadful, osteomyelitis with extension to the dura and subdural abscess or fatal meningitis.

2. *By partial removal of the orbital tissues,* which is commonly done when resecting localized, encapsulated orbital recurrences of intraocular malignant melanomas, retinoblastomas or some other neoplastic mesenchymal tumors. This has been called the subtotal exenteration [4]. Although it may be useful in some cases of recurrent malignant melanomas, where total exenteration may lessen the immunosuppressive cellular reactions, still it is not the soundest surgical recommendation.

3. *By partial or total preservation of eyelids* in an effort to obtain better cosmetic results. This can be performed in different manners: (a) Sever the eyelids just above the tarsal plates, to secure enough skin to close the orbital cavity in a tent-like manner. A pressure bandage helps to approximate the rough skin to the bare bone and the healing is rapid and uneventful. (b) Split the eyelids and, after removing the conjunctival portion, suture the eyelids together to close the orbital cavity. (c) In both previous cases the orbital cavity may be kept empty and only the organized clot would lessen the depth of the cavity, which soon can be fitted with a prosthesis [5]. (d) With partial preservation of both lids, the orbit can be immediately filled with: (1) temporalis muscle and its deep aponeurosis, as in Reese and Jones' [6] or Nankin's [7] techniques; (2) an orbital implant wrapped with buccal mucosa, as in Casanova's [8] technique; or (3) a pneumatic Salcedo [9] implant or an expandable Soll orbital implant, which may be filled with air in the former instance or with liquid Silastic in the latter.

Such variations lead to a common inconvenience: in concealing the prompt recognition of a local malignant recurrence, the patient is deprived of opportunities to be cured. The ophthalmologist must not overlook the fact that in dealing with malignant tumors, the cosmetic appearance after surgery is secondary to the chances of cure by radical excision of the malignancy.

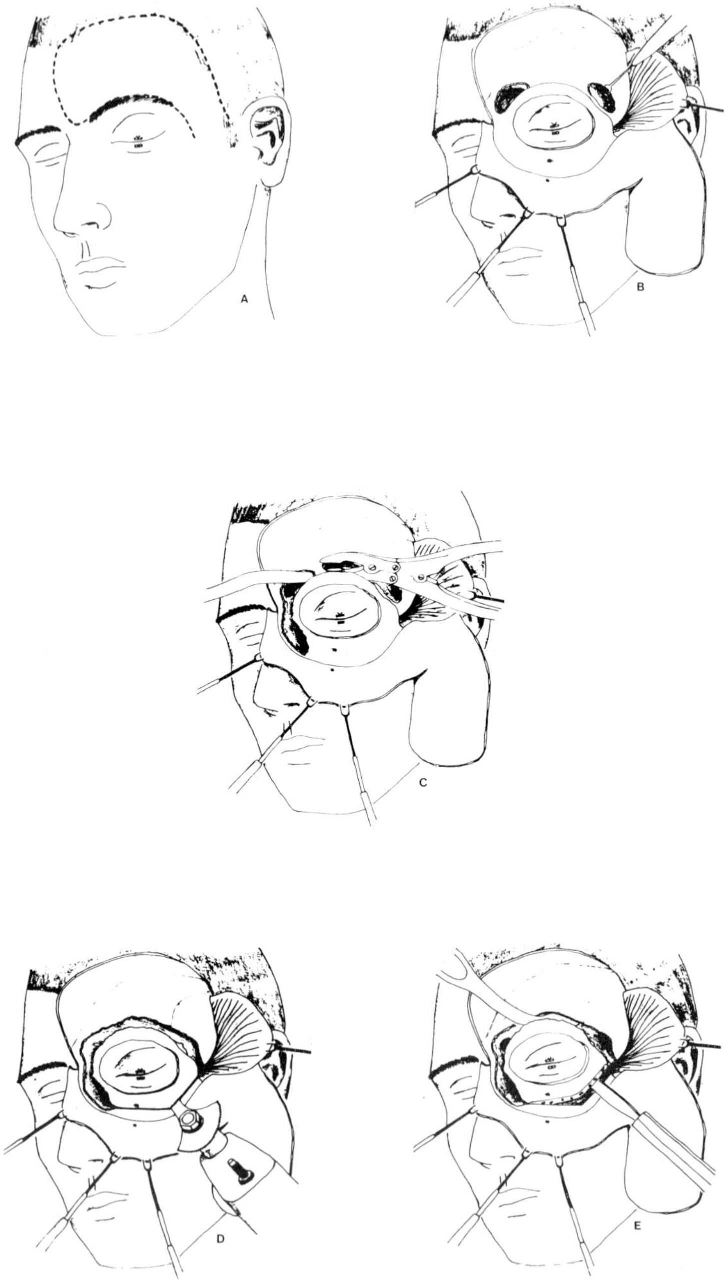
A
B
C
D
E

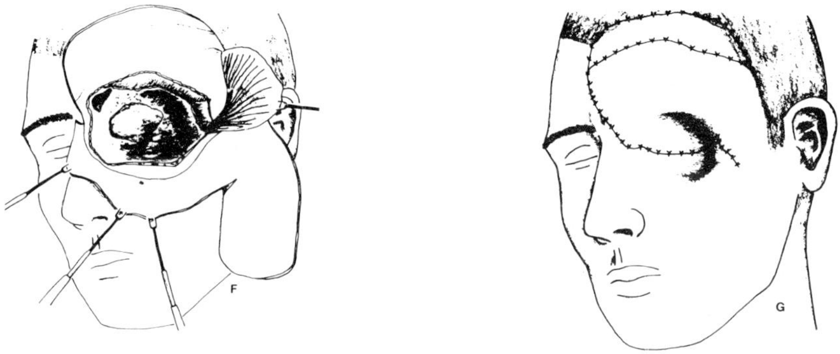

FIG. 2. Atypical orbital exenteration – enlarged exenteration with en bloc resection of the entire bony orbit (Barbosa's technique). (A) After the eyelids are sutured, the cutaneous flap is cut down to the periostium. The incision goes inside the hairline and passes downward slightly past the middle of the forehead, returning backward over the eyebrow as shown by the dotted line. (B) The cutaneous flap is reflected downward. The insertion of the temporalis muscle is severed and the temporal fossa denuded. A hole is trephined and the anterior cerebral fossa is exposed. If no tumor is found, a second hole is made on the posterior wall of the frontal sinus. (C) The entire superior side is sectioned with a rongeur, the dura being protected with a cerebral retractor. The incision is extended downward, resecting the entire ethmoidal sinus. (D) With a Stryker saw the inferior and lateral orbital rim is sectioned. (E) A malleable brain retractor is placed on the dura before fracturing the thin bone of the deep orbital cavity. The optic nerve and the apical stump are severed. (F) The entire bony orbit and its contents are resected. The dura of the anterior cranial fossa and a small part of the middle fossa can be seen, as well as both the optic foramen and the sphenoidal fissure. A great hole in the exposed nasal mucosa is seen medially. (G) The temporalis muscle is sutured as far anteriorly as possible to fill up the most external part of the orbital cavity. The skin flap is sutured after the sectioned and reflected periosteum of the frontal bone has been fixed to cover the exposed dura. A free skin graft is placed to fill the denuded area on the upper part of the forehead.

In a great number of cases a typical orbital exenteration will not be sufficient to eradicate the malignancy with wide margins of security. If the tumor invades the normal protective barrier, the periorbita, the subjacent bone must be resected to prevent recurrences. There is no limitation in superficial bone resections. The entire bony orbit can be resected en block if necessary (Fig. 2). But if tumor tissue is found infiltrating the dura, the surgery must not be continued [10].

The enlarged orbital exenteration can also be classified into different groups: (1) When the resection of the soft orbital tissues is complemented with *excision of invaded bony areas.* This is the most common type of exenteration in cases of tumors of the lacrimal gland [11], in eyelid or epibulbar carcinomas where the soft tissues are fixed to the orbital rim,

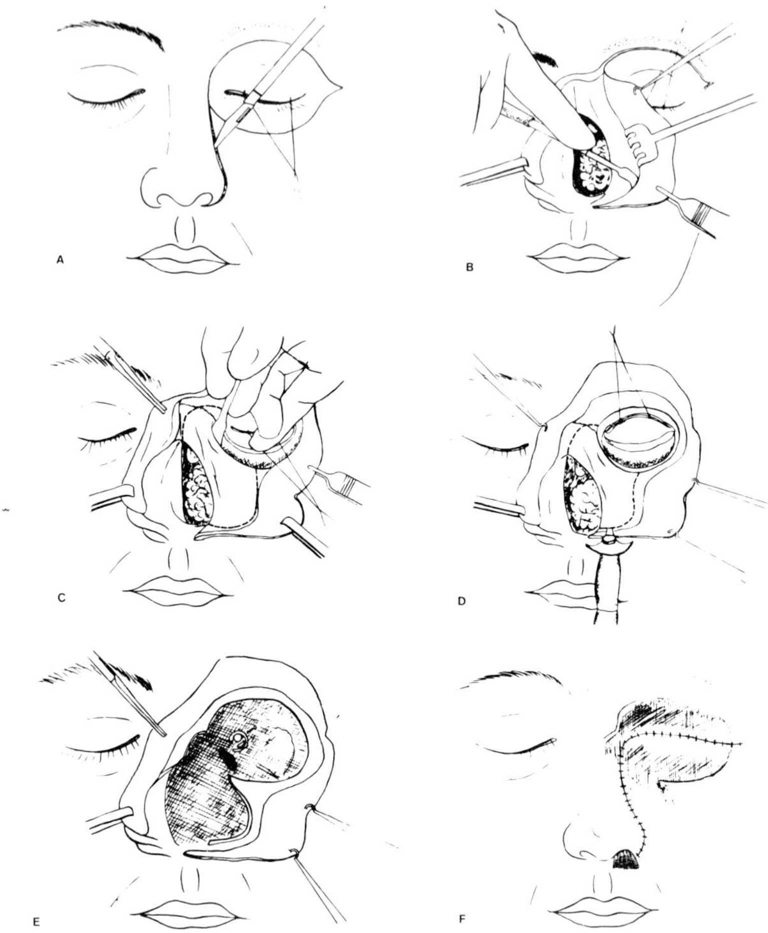

FIG. 3. Orbital exenteration with anterior rhinostomy. (A) The normal incision over the orbital rim is complemented with a lateral nasal incision that goes from the inner canthus to the base of the ala. The eyelids are sutured together and the sutures referred to a forceps to aid surgical maneuvers during the exenteration step. (B) The lateral soft tissues of the nose are severed. A skin flap is reflected laterally and the maxillary process, the nasal proper bones and the lacrimal bone are exposed. (C) The periosteum of the orbit is elevated up to the apical stump. The bone section is outlined. (D) The bone is severed with a Stryker saw and rongeur. The optic nerve and eye pedicle are sectioned and the pansinusectomy is performed. (E) A large naso-orbital cavity is left with extension to the paranasal sinus cavities, which have been curetted away. Gauze packing and fulguration aid to control the hemorrhagic oozing. (F) The bare cavity is filled with strips of gauze embedded in Furacin. The

cutaneous flap, with a split skin-graft lining is sutured back. A pressure bandage is placed over the naso-orbital area and left untouched for five days before removal for dressing. The nasal end of the gauze packing is pulled out on the first day; removal of the remainder is completed at the time of the first dressing.

---

etc. (2) When the orbital exenteration is complemented with *resection of the invaded sinus cavities* with or without anterior rhinostomy [12]. The invasion most frequently found is to the ethmoid and frontal sinuses in cases of basal cell carcinomas of the lid, and the maxillary antrum is more often affected in invasive squamous cell epibulbar or conjunctival carcinomas. (3) When the orbit has been invaded by rhinogenic tumors, *a partial or total maxillectomy* must complement the orbital exenteration. It is also common to perform such wide radical resections after irradiation treatments for undifferentiated tumors of paranasal cavities where residual tumor is found or eye and orbital tissues have been harmed. After maxillary resection, the cutaneous flap with a skin graft lining is sutured back and supported by a mold which reduces the cicatricial shrinkage. A week later an obturator prosthesis is placed over the palate to occlude the surgical communication between the mouth and the naso-orbital cavity, thus permitting normal feeding. The healing process is simple and the eye prosthesis can be adjusted in similar time as after a typical exenteration (Fig. 3).

As a rule, a well-performed orbital exenteration with immediate skin graft seldom presents important complications [13]. An eye prosthesis can be fitted early and cosmetic blemish is well concealed. Atypical techniques that tend to improve immediate cosmetic appearance are not justifiable on oncologic grounds. The healing time in an enlarged orbital exenteration may be prolonged, but its evolution parallels a typical one. The most common complications arise from the skin graft itself: excessive thickness, sloughing of the graft, devitalization after postoperative radiation, irregular adhesion due to uncontrolled hemorrhage or deep fulguration and, of course, infection of the graft and/or the subjacent bone. An important complication may occur in patients with previous neurosurgical orbital treatments. The dura is very easily torn during the surgical maneuvers and the graft takes very badly, thus increasing the chances of meningeal infection. Cerebral edema with orbital herniation is also a very distressing complication.

Minor nuisances may lead patients to disregard wearing the prosthesis: skin sensitivity to adhesives, discoloration of the plastic material, weight of the supporting frame, etc. In the long run, most patients return to wearing the black patch, to their doctors' disappointment.

Summary

Orbital exenteration is a radical surgical technique that must be reserved for the treatment of malignant diseases of the orbital region. The technique of a typical orbital exenteration is described, and the variations of the surgical procedure that change it into an atypical one are classified according to the surgeon's objectives: to minimize the surgical injury and improve the immediate cosmetic results, or to perform the radical excision of the malignancy with wide tumor-free margins. Both types of modifications are evaluated and their surgical and prosthetic complications are discussed.

References

1. Kirby, D.B.: Two cases of exenteration of the orbit with skin graft. Arch. Ophthal., 6:309-311, 1931.
2. Iliff, C. E.: Tumors of the orbit. Trans. Amer. Ophthal. Soc., 55:505-541, 1957.
3. Silva, D.: Orbital tumors. Amer. J. Ophthal., 65:318-339, 1968.
4. Henderson, J. W.: Orbital Tumors. Philadelphia:W. B. Saunders Co. 1973, p. 662.
5. Fuchs, A.: Simple last steps of exenteratio orbitae. Arch. Ophthal., 55:692-693, 1956.
6. Jones, I.: Unilateral exophthalmos. Highlights Ophthal., 1-79, 1963.
7. Nankin, H.: Orbital reconstruction utilizing temporalis muscle. Amer. J. Ophthal., 41:519-521, 1956.
8. Casanova, J. and Mir y Mir, L.: Perfeccionamientos en al evisceración orbitaria. Arch. Soc. Oftal. Hisp. Amer., 19:249-260, 1959.
9. Salcedo, M.: El problema cosmético de la exenteración orbitaria. Arch. APEC México, 49:48-57, 1968.
10. Barbosa, J. F.: Surgical Treatment of Head and Neck Tumors. New York.Grune & Stratton Inc., 1974.
11. Reese, A. B. and Jones, I. S.: Bone resection in the excision of epithelial tumors of the lacrimal gland. Arch. Ophthal., 71:382-385, 1964.
12. Conley, J.: Concepts in Head and Neck Surgery. New York:Grune & Stratton Inc., 1970.
13. Iliff, C. E.: Complications of exenteration of the orbit. *In* Fasanella, R. M. (ed.): Complications in Eye Surgery. Philadelphia:W. B. Saunders Co., 1965, pp. 426-432.

Congenital Deformities: Maturation in Microorbit and Microphthalmos

Vernon R. Lamb

How can the ocularist and the ophthalmologist better correct the congenital deformities of microorbit and microphthalmos? Numerous authors have discussed the maturation of the congenital orbital-socket deformity seen in microorbit and microphthalmos. I have used all their methods with a few gratifying results. To achieve a more satisfying end result requires newer and more efficient methods.

One feels most frustrated when years of continuous effort on these sockets do not produce a desirable cosmetic result – one which would allow the patient to go through life with psychological security and comfort.

The following letter, I feel certain, describes the experience of everyone in the field. It is a response from an ophthalmologist upon request for a summary. In addition to the ophthalmologist's efforts, we have seen this girl many times. Often we did not know which way to proceed in assisting growth of socket, lids and orbit.

> The following is a summary of my record on patient X. She was first seen February 25, 1965, at age one with a history of having had an enucleation by an ophthalmologist in Fort Worth some six months prior for a retinoblastoma. She was wearing a prosthesis which I understood you had fitted. Left eye was negative. She was followed rather closely by both myself and the ophthalmologist for the first couple of years with respect to the left eye and for recurrence in the socket.
>
> I have a history here that you saw her January 1967 and again in July and had observed what they described as lid trouble. This was the shortening of the lid. By this time she really had almost no lower lid. She never really had a frank socket infection although she had

Vernon R. Lamb, F.C.L.S.A., Ocularist, San Angelo, Texas.

the usual mucoid drainage. April 4, 1970, I did a Z-plasty and some other reconstruction in the socket, mainly to reduce the tight band of fibrous tissue from the lid at 2 o'clock to the implant. A large conformer was placed in the cul-de-sac and the lids were sutured together, using a single double arm #0000 black silk. This helped some but really nothing dramatic resulted from the surgery. July 18, 1972, a large granuloma was excised from the socket.

The course of this condition through the years is remarkable in the progressive loss of the lower lid and inferior cul-de-sac, progressing finally to inability to retain the prosthesis. Some time in January, 1974, the ophthalmologist in Fort Worth did a reconstruction of the socket, and she was wearing your pressurized lid conformer when I saw her. She looked good for a time, but by the middle of February most of the improvement had been lost to the point of inability to retain the conformer again. The last time I saw her was March 18, 1974, following a visit to you. At that time she seemed to have a little more room in the cul-de-sac but still had marked socket contraction. Hope this is of some help to you.

This letter demonstrates numerous setbacks, repetitive surgery and prosthetics, all with generally poor results in socket development. Where do we go from here? Did we do the things we should, could or would have done if the ophthalmologist-ocularist team did more work?

The same general problems arise in all such cases. First, the normal bony socket will not develop without retaining the pathologic globe as long as possible in childhood [1]. Removal demands some type of implantation followed by a regular, continuous program of corrective prosthetics [2]. These include progressively enlarged conformers or pressure conformers as described by S. S. Kelly [3], Fritz Jardon [4], H. Gougelmann, et al. Expandable conformers are also a convenient form of pressure in the cul-de-sac and offer a versatile method of home therapy [5]. These prosthetics work to some degree, but finally surgical intervention is required to enhance socket development [6].

As described in the letter, there usually is continual loss of the cul-de-sacs with lower lid entropion developing [7]. Due to continual restriction and absence of normal secretion drainage, blepharitis of the socket causes loss of lower lashes and facial tissue scarring [8]. Pressures of the prosthetic usually attack the upper tarsal plate, causing a bending in the middle which allows no filling of the upper fold. Abnormal temporal arching of the upper lid results. This restriction does not allow for stretching of the conjunctiva through exercise.

Sockets forced in depth to the posterior walls of the orbit become very unsightly. When we seek to achieve forward movement of the lids and adnexa as growth occurs, we must concentrate on pressures circumscribed about the cul-de-sacs, rather than pushing deeper [9]. Backward pressure must be kept balanced and uniform over a broad surface to eliminate extrusion of the implants.

When surgery becomes necessary to reconstruct the socket, a mucoid graft is preferable. Skin grafts lack motility and create serious hygiene problems. I have observed after surgical procedures to stretch the lids that removal of sutures even after four to six weeks allows prolapsing of the socket despite pressure bandages, dumbbell conformers, etc. A longer period before removing sutures might help.

Even more, some type of upper and lower lid attachment similar to orthodontic bands attached to wires following the upper and lower lid margins, then laced together like bootlaces, could help stretch the tissue without causing entropion and restriction. Physical therapy by tugging on the lashes only causes more tissue inflammation, loss of lashes and little result compared to effort exerted.

In all these cases we need to follow the patient more closely and make alterations of the prosthetic attachments more frequently. Removal of the prosthesis by accident or upon instruction by the ophthalmologist for cleaning has caused complete loss of upper and lower cul-de-sacs in many cases. In some cases, to keep the simplest conformer in place required more surgery. Sometimes years of effort were lost.

I do not recommend removal of any prosthesis for cleaning when normal lid closure can be accomplished, except for periodic resurfacing or inspection by the ophthalmologist. In restricted sockets and skin grafts this removal should be brief. If there is any chance of the patient or guardians not being able to maintain the prosthetic device in the socket, then even daily hygiene should be performed by the ocularist. In most cases this is impractical.

Maturation of the congenital orbital-socket deformity is a long, continual process with many of the same difficulties arising in each case. These include loss of the upper and lower cul-de-sacs causing entropion, loss of lashes and restriction of both lid function and mobility. As many other contributors point out, the normal globe should be retained as long as feasible, while corrective prosthetics must be applied continually. Mucoid grafting is much preferred to skin grafting. The greatest problem is maintenance of the forward position of the prosthesis together with lid and facial conformation.

The patient used as this paper's example (Figs. 1-10) was also seen recently for consultation by another practitioner. His response emphasizes the basic purpose of this paper as follows:

> Thank you very much for referring patient X. I saw her on June 12, 1974 and did careful measurements and photographs of her eyes. I think you have done a fine job with your expanding prosthesis. I do not think anything more can be done along this line. However, there is some possibility that we may be able to do some orbital surgery. What is needed is something to bring the upper and lower lids and prosthesis forward as a unit, since there is marked enophthalmos.
>
> I have not completely made a decision on this case and will be in touch with you at a later time.

Solving the problems of microorbit and microphthalmos requires a definite team effort between the ocularist and ophthalmologist. The important future question remains, where do we go from here? I challenge both the ophthalmologist and the ocularist to work in the development of new and better prosthetics and therapeutic procedures to solve this problem.

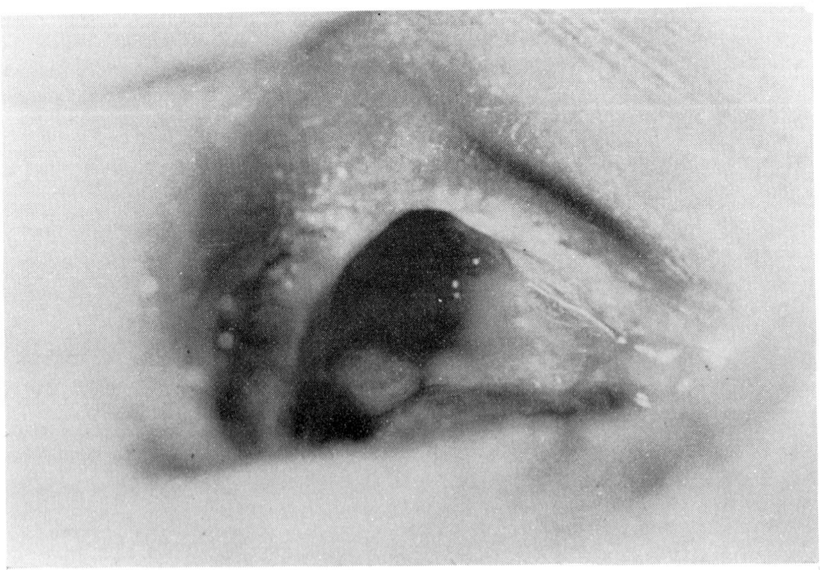

FIG. 1. Socket prior to mucoid graft. Note very poor upper cul-de-sac and shortening of both upper and lower lids and cul-de-sacs.

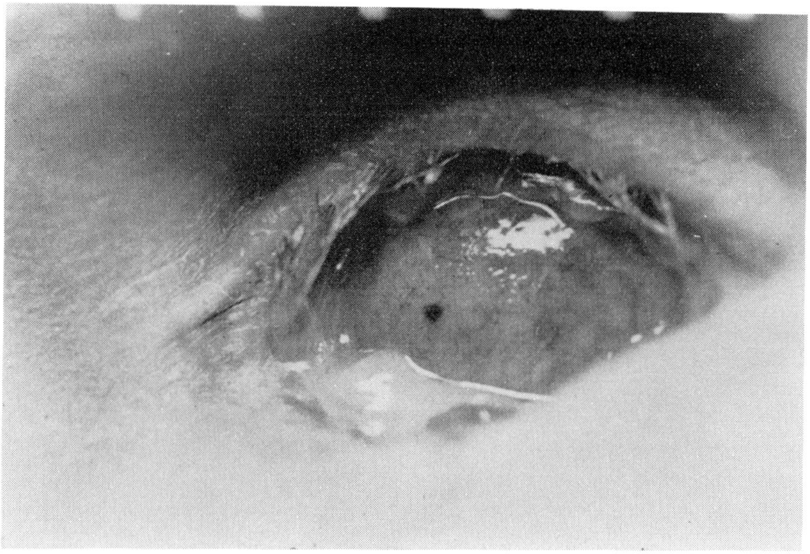

FIG. 2. Forward movement of the old implant after mucoid grafting. Note mucoid palp on lower temporal cul-de-sac.

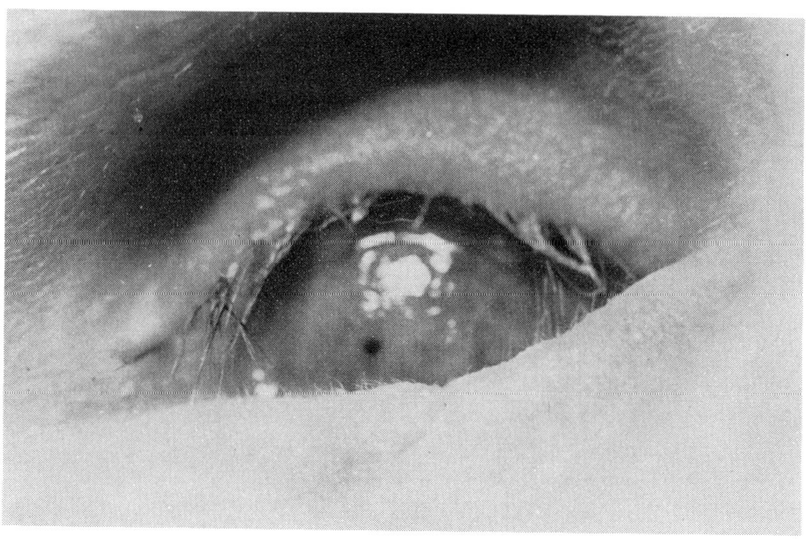

FIG. 3. Socket results after use of dumbbell conformers with pressure bandages and expandable prosthetics.

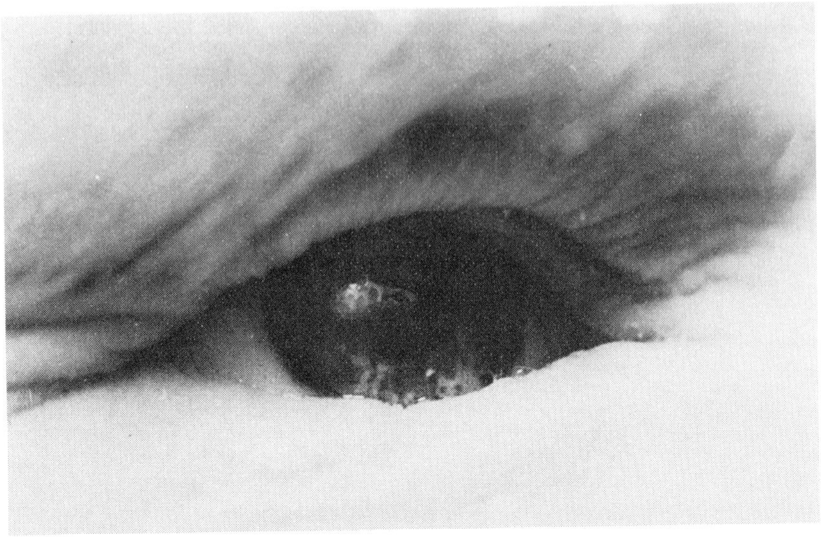

FIG. 4. Patient during a squeezing-type exercise at home. Note the severe restriction of upper and lower lids and basic entropion of both. At this stage actually more stretching of the outer skin tissue takes place than the needed stretching of the conjunctiva in the socket.

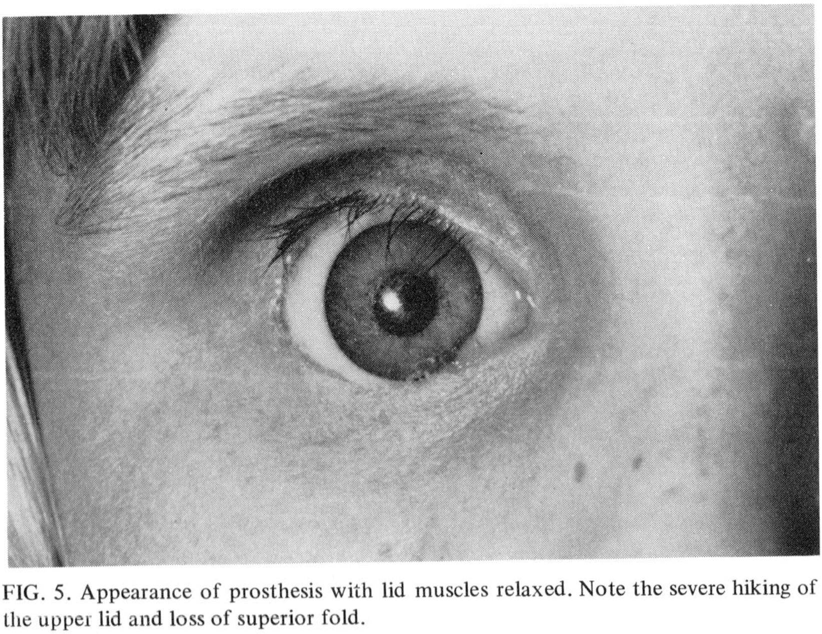

FIG. 5. Appearance of prosthesis with lid muscles relaxed. Note the severe hiking of the upper lid and loss of superior fold.

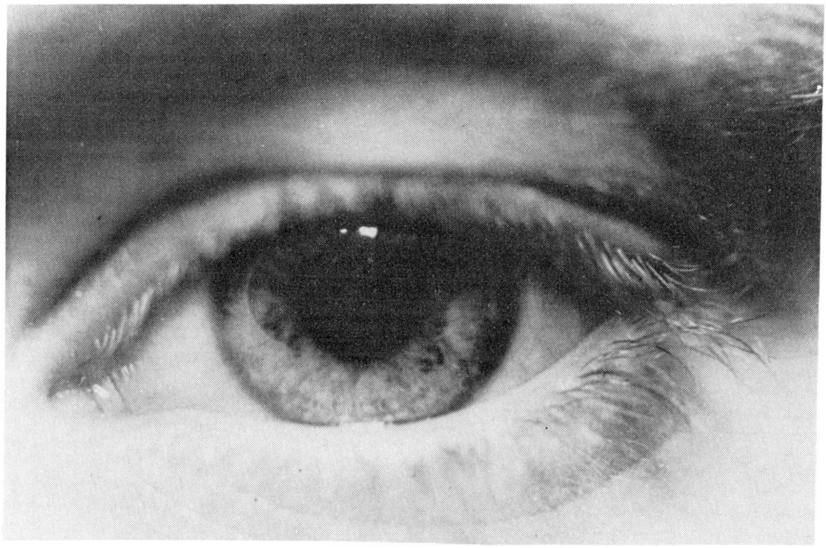

FIG. 6. Patient's normal eye under same magnification as Figure 4.

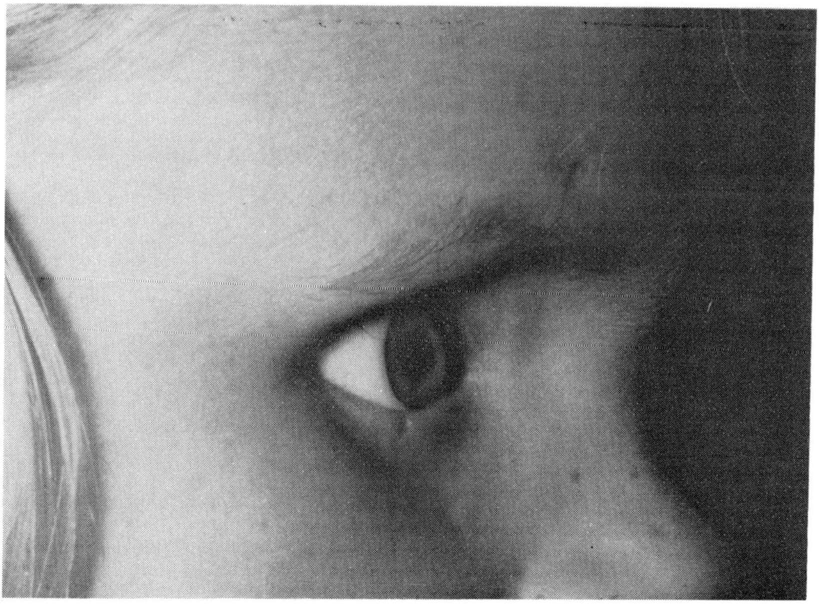

FIG. 7. The prosthetic eye at cross section to the face; note the sunken appearance.

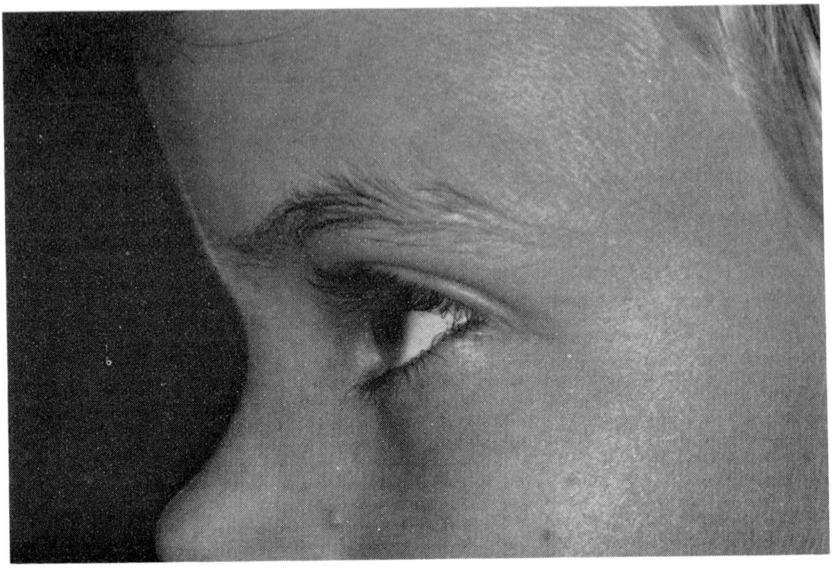

FIG. 8. The normal eye. Note the forward positioning of the upper lid and lower cheek area.

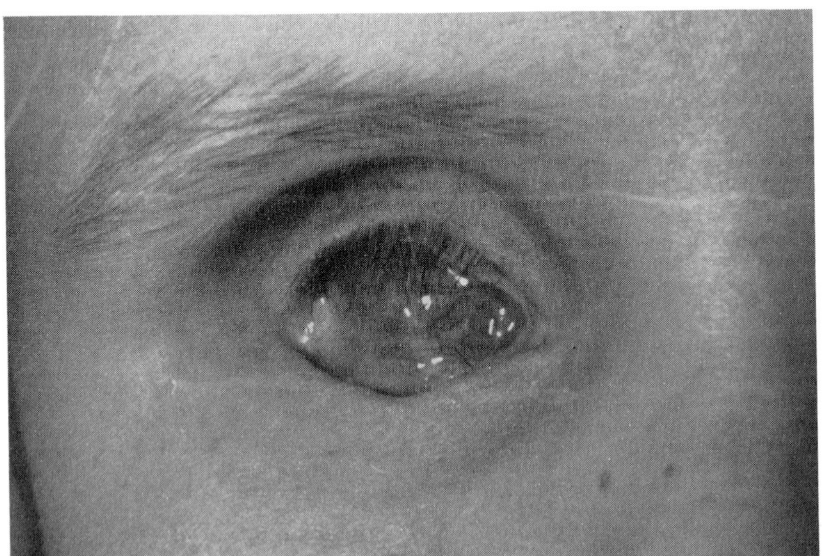

FIG. 9. The empty socket after approximately nine months of therapy with the existing prosthesis.

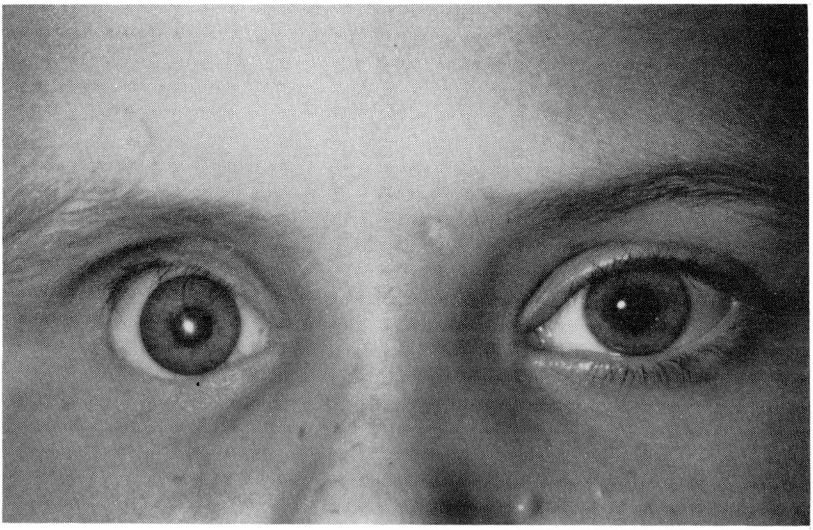

FIG. 10. Present cosmetic result comparison.

References

1. Guibor, P.: Contracted sockets – Statement of problems and treatment. *In* Guibor, P. and Gougelmann, H. (eds.): Problems and Treatment of Contracted Sockets, Exenterated Orbits, Alkali Burns. Miami:Symposia Specialists, 1973, vol. 1, pp. 11-22.
2. Spaeth, E. B.: Shrunken socket and related orbital hypoplasia (surgical correction). *In* Shannon and Connelly (eds.): Oculoplastic Surgery and Prosthetics. Boston:Little, Brown & Co., 1970, vol. 10C, no. 4, pp. 879-895.
3. Workman, C. L.: Loss of inferior cul-de-sac (prosthetic correction). *In* Shannon and Connelly (eds.): Oculoplastic Surgery and Prosthetics. Boston:Little, Brown & Co., vol. 10C, no. 4, pp. 835-840.
4. Kelley, J. J.: Contraction of the anophthalmic orbit – Statement of the problem and prosthetic treatment. *In* Guibor, P. and Gougelmann, H. (eds.): Problems and Treatment of Contracted Sockets, Exenterated Orbits, Alkali Burns. Miami: Symposia Specialists, 1973, vol. 1, pp. 3-9.
5. Jardon, F.: Prostheses for the contracted socket. *In* Guibor, P. and Gougelmann, H. (eds.): Problems and Treatment of Contracted Sockets, Exenterated Orbits, Alkali Burns. Miami:Symposia Specialists, vol. 1, pp. 23-28.
6. Soll, D. B., Frisch, E. and Asbell, R. L.: Congenital anophthalmos – Experimental devices in socket expansion. *In* Guibor, P. and Gougelmann, H. (eds.): Problems and Treatment of Contracted Sockets, Exenterated Orbits, Alkali Burns. Miami:Symposia Specialists, vol. 1, pp. 43-49.
7. Flanagan, J. C.: Loss of the lower cul-de-sac (surgical technique). *In* Shannon and Connelly (eds.): Oculoplastic Surgery and Prosthetics. Boston:Little, Brown &

Co., 1970, vol. 10C, no. 4, pp. 825-833.

8. Mulberger, R. D.: Trauma with lid deformities (surgical correction). *In* Shannon and Connelly (eds.): Oculoplastic Surgery and Prosthetics. Boston:Little, Brown & Co., 1970, vol. 10C, no. 4, pp. 874-876.
9. Barr, D.: The dumbbell pressure conformer. *In* Guibor, P. and Gougelmann, H. (eds.): Problems and Treatment of Contracted Sockets, Exenterated Orbits, Alkali Burns. Miami:Symposia Specialists, 1973, vol. 1, pp. 29-36.

Influence of the Ocularist and Ophthalmologist in Microorbit and Microphthalmos

Robert G. Small, M.D. and Edward Dalton, M.D.

When a child is born with no eye or with a small or rudimentary eye and adnexa, the distraught parents will soon seek medical attention. They want a normal appearance. If an eye is present they want to know if there is usable vision. The ophthalmic plastic surgeon is presented with the problem of abnormalities in the soft tissue of the adnexa of the eye as well as the bony orbit. He must determine whether there is any possible function in the abnormal eye. He must also rule out the possiblity of tumor.

The problems in treatment include a socket too small for a prosthesis, abnormal lid function, possible irritation of the microphthalmic eye by the prosthesis which rides over it, the decision as to whether to utilize plastic surgery or orbital expanders in treatment, and the possiblity of prolonged treatment and repeated anesthesia.

Pathology

Complete anophthalmos is rare and usually bilateral. Unilateral microphthalmos is more frequent with either a rudimentary sightless eye or a small eye with little or no usable vision. The lids and adnexa are also often small and abnormal. Lid function may be reduced or absent. The bony orbit is usually smaller than the normal orbit. There may be asymmetry of the face and other congenital defects.

Robert G. Small, M.D. Clinical Associate Professor of Ophthalmology; and Edward Dalton, M.D., Clinical Instructor, Division of Plastic Surgery, Health Sciences Center, University of Oklahoma, Oklahoma City.

Treatment

The use of early surgery in microphthalmos will be discussed in *Case 1*, in which multiple surgeries were carried out. The use of nonoperative treatment with expanders will be discussed in *Case 2*.

Case 1. An 11-year-old boy was first seen by the author in November 1971 at age 8. Either no eye or a rudimentary eye was present at birth. He had had at least 12 procedures on his microphthalmic right orbit before I saw him (Fig. 1). Some of these were attempts to use orbital expanders. Others were attempts at surgical orbital reconstruction. The first procedure had been carried out at age 7 months. Details of the operations were not available. He was unable to wear a prosthesis and was using a black patch. The mother and patient were very cooperative and anxious for a suitable cosmetic appearance. Five additional operations were done. Two of these were extensive. There has been success in that the patient is now able to wear a prosthesis and prefers this to the use of a patch.

The first procedure by me, in May 1972 (the 13th operation on the patient), was an orbital reconstruction with split-thickness skin graft. The graft was wrapped around a plastic conformer and placed in the orbit in the hope of creating fornices which would enable the patient to wear a prosthesis. This resulted in only slight enlargement of the socket and no significant increase in the depth of the fornices.

On April 17, 1973, he had a Z-plasty of the right eyebrow, a buried dermal bridge and skin flap, a composite graft of skin and cartilage from the ear into the upper and lower fornix [1], a full-thickness postauricular skin graft to the donor defect in the right ear, a full-thickness postauricular skin graft to the eye socket, and an extensive dissection of the fornices and excision of remnants of the conjunctiva.

On July 10, 1973, cartilage grafts were taken from the left ear and placed in the fornices. A Z-plasty was done to raise the medial brow. Another Z-plasty was done to lower the lateral canthus. The right lower lid was defatted and an inverted "V" flap was carried out to enlarge the lateral fornix. Later a right lateral canthoplasty and revision of the right upper eyelid were done.

On August 20, 1974, a lateral tarsorrhaphy decreased the size of the gaping lateral canthus. This extensive surgical program has resulted in some success in terms of a fair cosmetic appearance (Fig. 2). The ocularist was present when necessary in the operating room. His working closely with the ophthalmologist was helpful in this case.

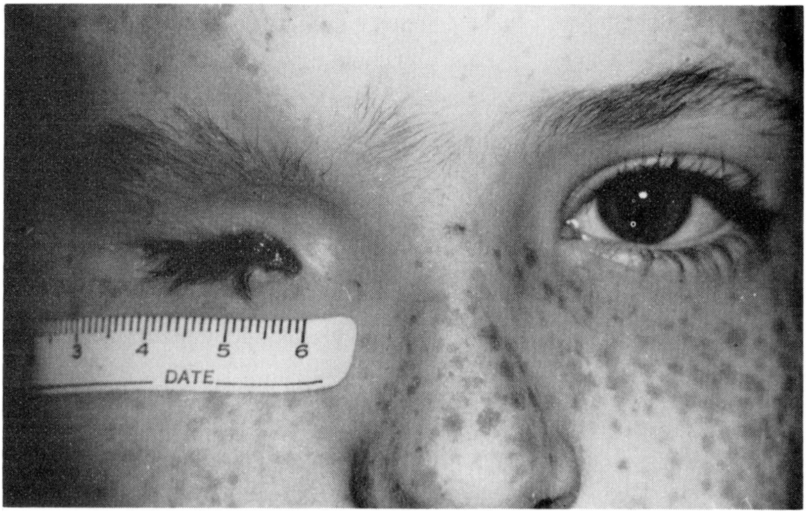

FIG. 1. *Case 1* at age 8 after 12 surgical procedures.

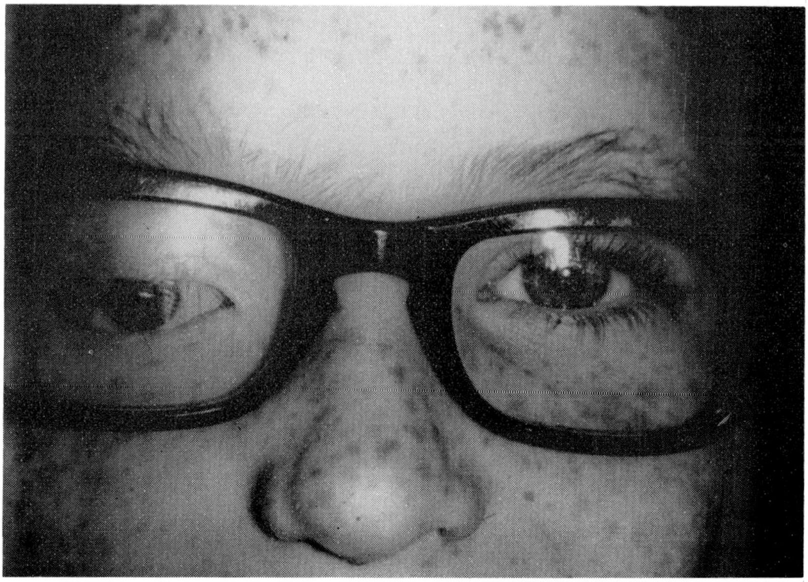

FIG. 2. *Case 1,* final result.

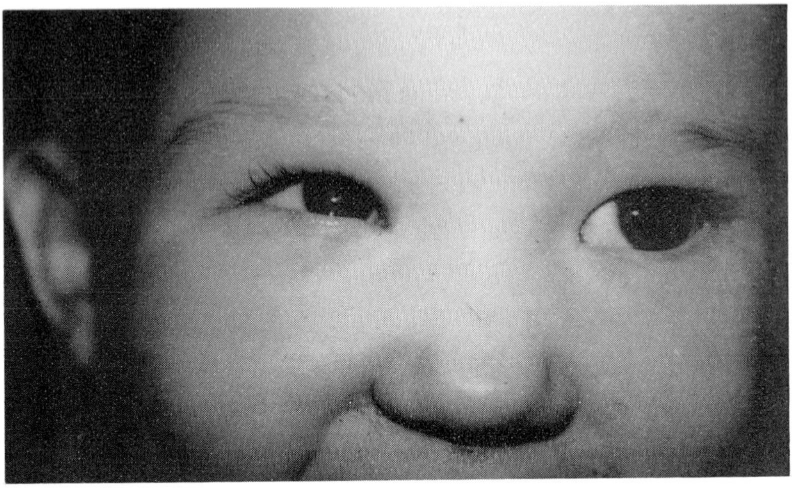

FIG. 3. *Case 2* prior to treatment.

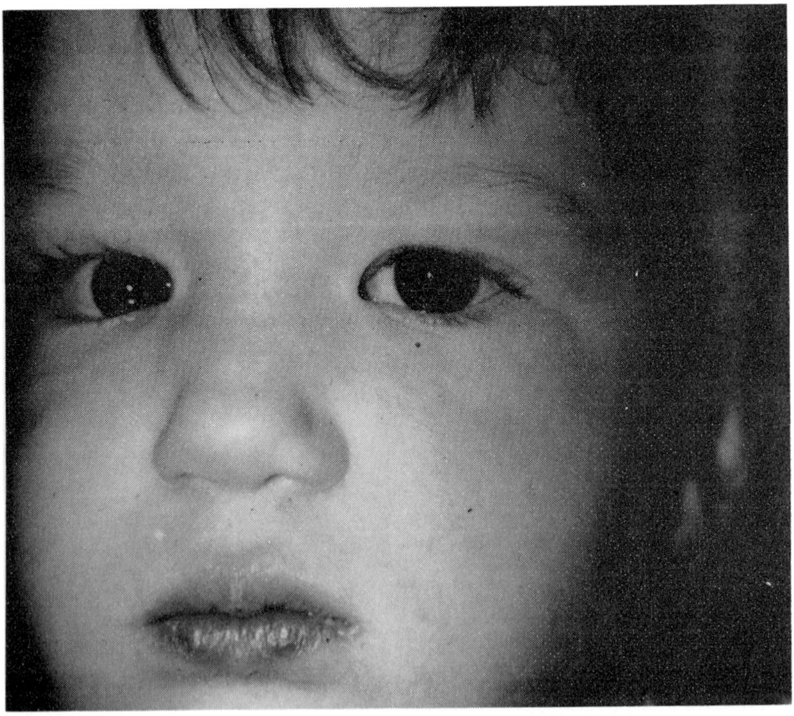

FIG. 4. *Case 2* after use of expanders.

Case 2. A 2-year-old white girl was born with a small right eye (Fig. 3). No surgical treatment was instituted and progressive expanders were placed in the orbit under general anesthesia. After treatment for one year the patient can wear a prosthesis with a satisfactory cosmetic appearance (Fig. 4). A conjunctival flap was done because of irritation of the microphthalmic eye by the prosthesis. This case is not completely comparable to *Case 1* since the microphthalmos and microorbit are not as severe. As in *Case 1*, the ophthalmologist and ocularist worked closely together. The final impression for the prosthesis was taken under anesthesia in the operating room by the ocularist.

Discussion

The early procedures carried out in *Case 1* make one wonder whether a better result might have been obtained if surgery had been deferred until late childhood. It is possible that a small eye was enucleated early in the treatment. As Robert Kennedy of Rochester has shown [2], early enucleation has a definite effect in retarding the growth of the orbit. *Case 1* suggests that repeated orbital surgery in an infant or young child is likely to be unsuccessful. The utmost caution should be exercised in embarking on orbital soft tissue surgery early in life.

If surgery is elected, one should wait until the child is at an age when most of the growth of the eye and orbit has taken place. Even then, one should be prepared to employ extensive grafting procedures with the use of skin grafts, cartilage grafts, Z-plasty, tunnel flaps and other plastic surgical maneuvers where indicated, since simple orbital reconstruction with a mucous membrane or skin graft is not likely to be successful in children with microphthalmos.

Conclusion

The preceding cases underline principles which apply to orbital surgery early in life: (1) Do not enucleate eyes in infants or children, even if they are abnormally small, unless forced to do so because of tumor, pain or other urgent considerations. (2) Avoid the use of plastic surgical procedures in infants and young children in an attempt to enlarge the orbit and adnexa, particularly during the rapid growth period in the first few years of life. (3) Employ orbital expanders early in life and replace these at appropriate intervals under anesthesia. (4) The ocularist and ophthalmic plastic surgeon should work closely together. It is often desirable for the ocularist to be present in the operating room for impressions or when expanders and a prosthesis are being placed with the patient under anesthesia.

References

1. Orticochea, M.: Eye socket reconstruction with composite grafts. Plast. Reconstr. Surg., 48:343-346, Oct. 1971.
2. Kennedy, R. E.: The effect of early enucleation on the orbit in animals and humans. Amer. J. Ophthal., 60:277-306, Aug. 1965.

Influence of Congenital Deformities on Orbital Socket Maturation and Contracted Socket Repair

Robert E. Kennedy, M.D.

Concerning congenital deformities of the orbit, Dr. Robert Small cites a case of one eye which had 12 operative procedures prior to his seeing the patient, together with 5 of his own, for a total of 17 [1].

Two cases are to be presented in support of Dr. Small's presentation. One emphasizes the conservative approach, short of surgery in the anophthalmic orbit, where possible. The second case emphasizes radical, rather than minimal surgery where socket reconstruction is indicated.

Case Reports

Congenital Anophthalmos, Bilateral

Animal work has proved that in early enucleation the small orbit will show marked bone changes, as demonstrated in the cat [2]. Figure 1 shows these marked changes in the orbit when the right eye has been enucleated at less than 2 weeks of age and the skull allowed to mature to full growth; note the constriction on the left side of the picture. These changes may show decreased measurements in the magnitude of 25% to 30%. The same can be demonstrated (Fig. 2) in the human skull [3], where the decrease in the measurements is approximately 25% in the entrance to the orbit and 12% in the depth of the orbit, with the volume reduced by a remarkable 60% from an average 30 cc to a mere 12 cc. It is exceedingly rare to have the opportunity to make this study on human skulls except by x-ray evaluation, which is demonstrated in Figure 3, where the right orbit (left side of the picture) of a child under anesthesia demonstrates a much smaller shrunken orbit with overhanging rims and

---

Robert E. Kennedy, M.D., Clinical Professor of Ophthalmology, University of Rochester School of Medicine and Dentistry, Rochester, N. Y.

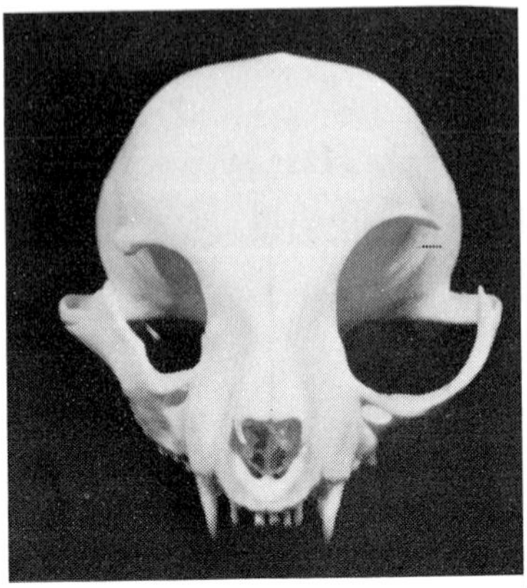

FIGURE 1.

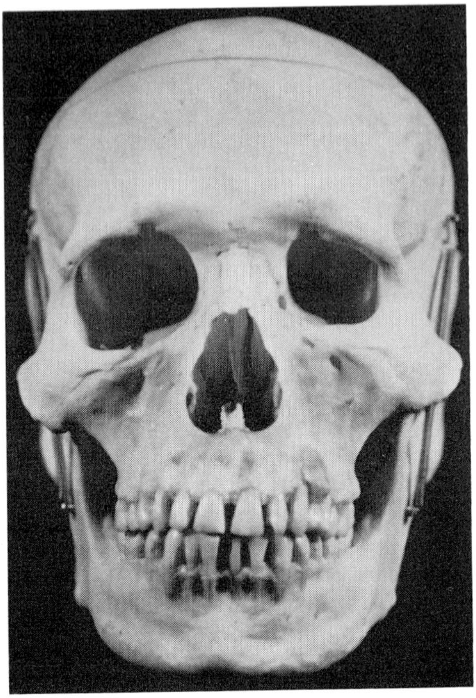

FIGURE 2.

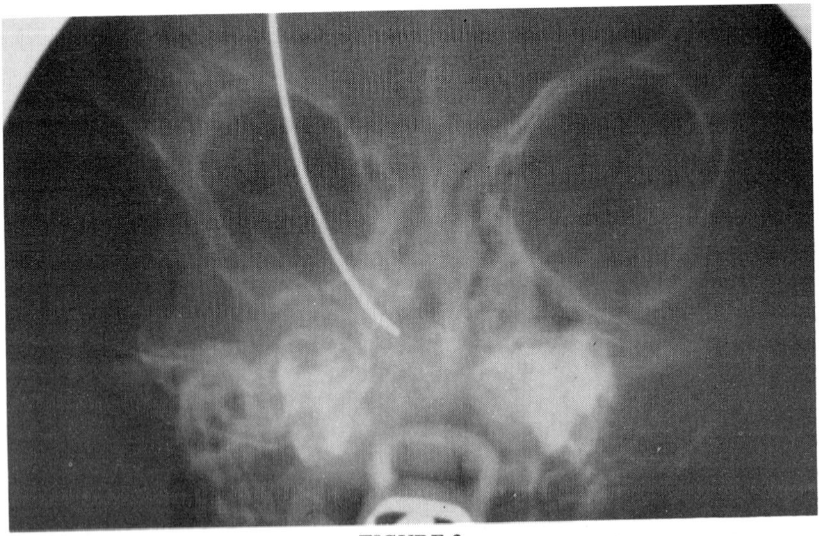

FIGURE 3.

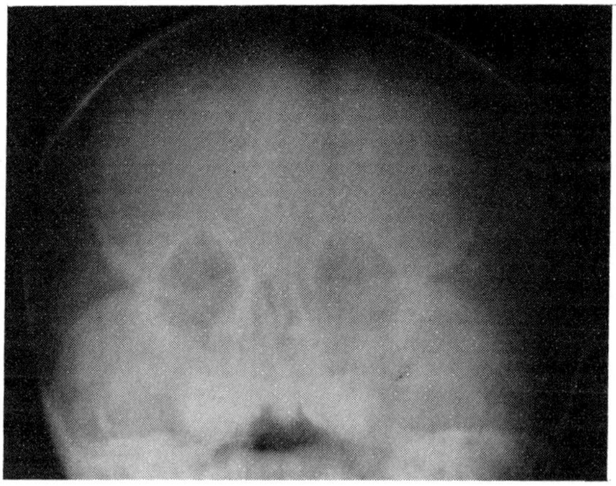

FIGURE 4.

irregular walls. Figure 4 reveals the dramatic changes of the tiny orbits as seen in a bilateral congenital anophthalmic patient.

Case 1. Figure 5 shows a 1-month-old patient born with bilateral anophthalmos, shrunken sockets and a pinched-together appearance of the face. At age 4 weeks, silicone rubber spheres (6 mm in size in the right socket and 7 mm in the left socket) were put in place and taped in position. At two- to three-week intervals these were increased in size from the standpoint of the spheres and gradually transferred to an oval button and then a mushroom-type prosthesis which was eventually covered with a conformer. These various devices are shown in Figure 6. A contact lens suction cup, or muscle hook, and local anesthetic will readily remove these prostheses. It is not necessary for the child to be put to sleep, with the annoyance of hospital admission and general anesthetic, if one has enough office assistance.

Figure 7 shows the child at age 7 months; and Figure 8 shows the child at 13 months, appearing quite normal, wearing prostheses measuring 18 by 23 mm with a depth of 18 mm in the shape of a mushroom. These prostheses will be increased in size as needed, and surgery and anesthesia have been avoided.

Approximately 75% of such patients can be handled medically if treatment is started extremely early, within the first month of life, thus avoiding the necessity for surgery. The size of the socket is more important than the size of the orbit. The orbit will remain smaller. An implant does increase the size of the orbit if placed at the time of enucleation [2], if enucleation is indicated, but does not benefit enough

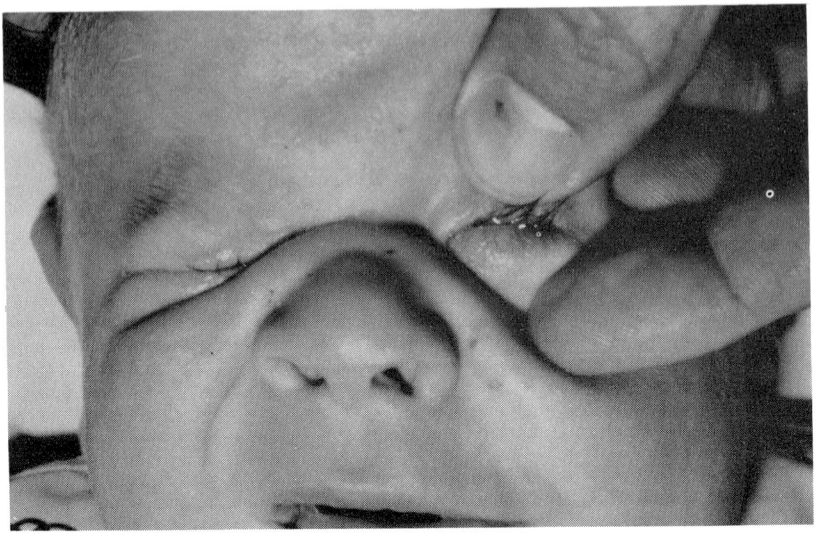

FIGURE 5.

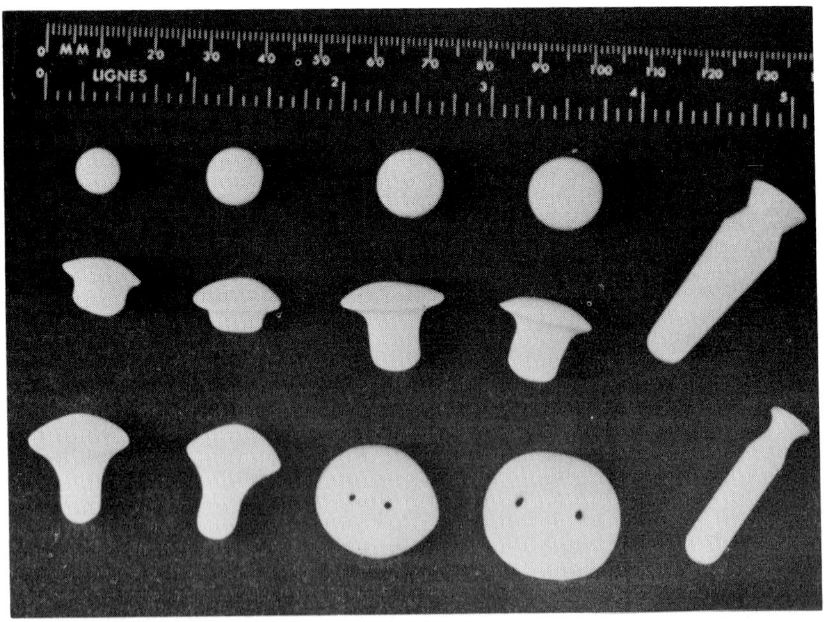

FIGURE 6.

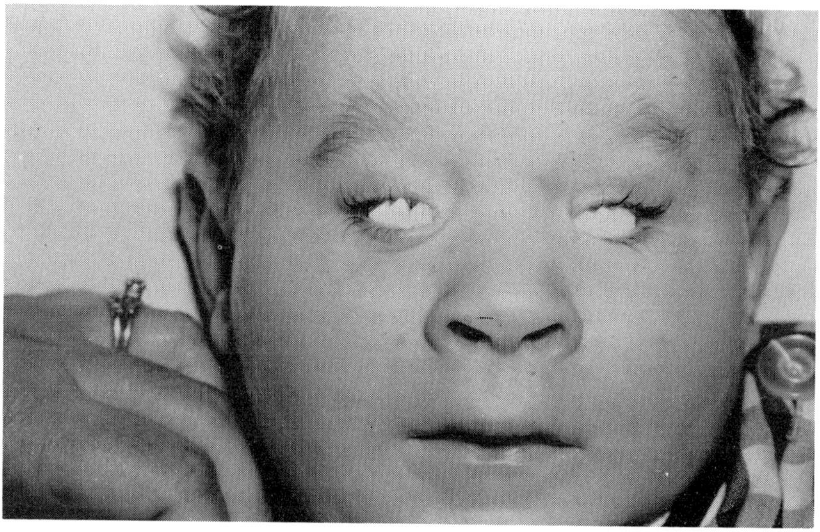

FIGURE 7.

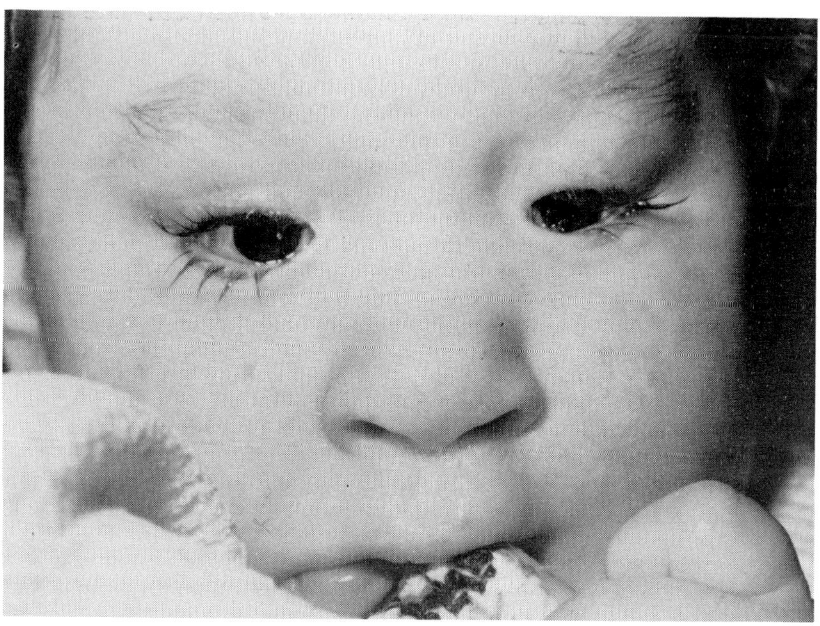

FIGURE 8.

to be used as a primary procedure in congenital anophthalmos. Surgery can only lead to scar tissue, bleeding and orbital fat atrophy. Deferring management, with the idea of radical bone resection at a later age with probable excision of conjunctiva and replacement with skin, is to be condemned. Very early conservative management is indicated in the first month of life.

Late Repair of the Grossly Contracted Socket

One of the most formidable procedures in ophthalmic plastic surgery is the repair of the grossly contracted socket. The previously cited case (Small [1]) illustrates that 12 minor "pecking away" procedures reduced the socket to the inability to wear a prosthesis, requiring 5 subsequent procedures before a satisfactory prosthesis could be worn. One must really "think big" in doing a surgical repair of such a socket.

The following case report is that of a patient illustrating the point of having a fairly radical procedure, which in itself was not extensive enough and required still an even more radical operation to solve her problem.

Case 2. A 42-year-old woman had been wearing an integrated implant for several years, with inability to wear a prosthesis for five years. This was ultimately removed followed by severe contracture of the socket. The contracted socket is shown in Figure 9. Holes were drilled through the inferior rim of the orbit (Fig. 10) so that a conformer, surrounded with mucous membrane taken from the mouth, could be wired into the operated socket to maintain its position and resist scar tissue. Figure 11 shows the patient 11 days following surgery with the lids sutured together. No tarsorrhaphy, however, should be performed. These usually break down from infection and disrupt the cosmesis of the lid margin. Following removal of the sutures on the 15th day (Fig. 12) the prosthesis looked very satisfactory. However, by six weeks (Fig. 13), the socket reveals the effects of the fierce contracture of the scar tissue which is continual, relentless and remorseless to the point of retracting the upper lid over the top of the large conformer, necessitating a further operative procedure.

Four months later a second procedure was performed using the principles encouraged by Callahan [4]. Figure 14 shows a very large conformer which was to be wired to the upper and lower rims of the orbit both nasally and temporally. The importance of a complete resection of all the underlying scar tissue when preparing the graft bed can not be emphasized too strongly. A large adequate graft,

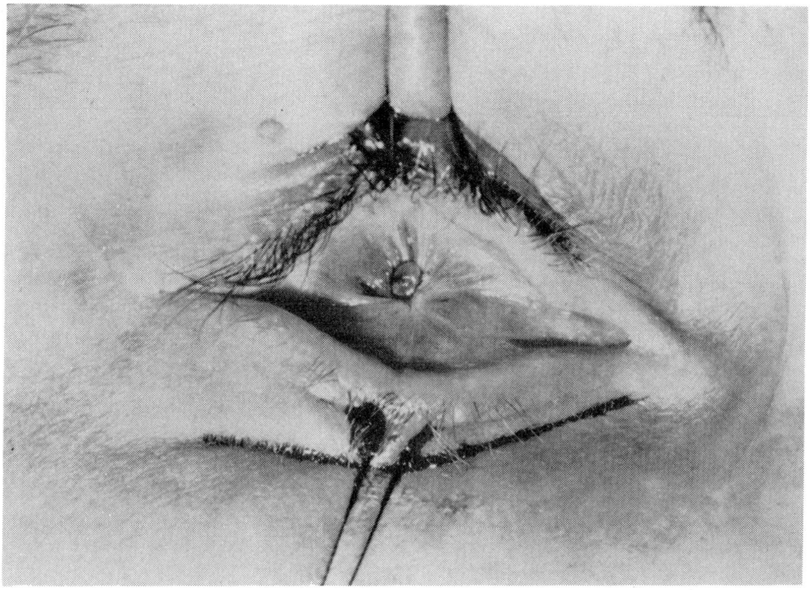

FIGURE 9.

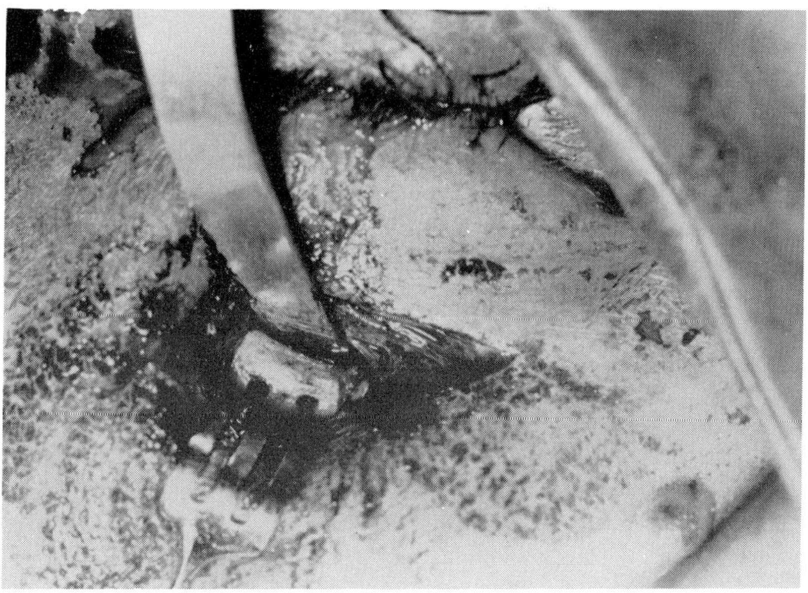

FIGURE 10.

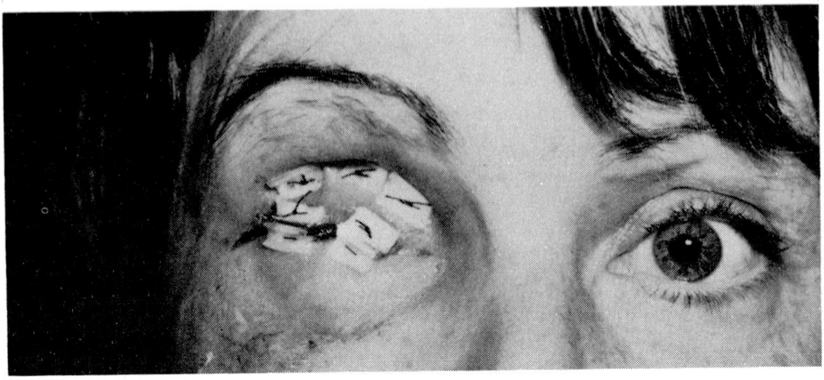

FIGURE 11.

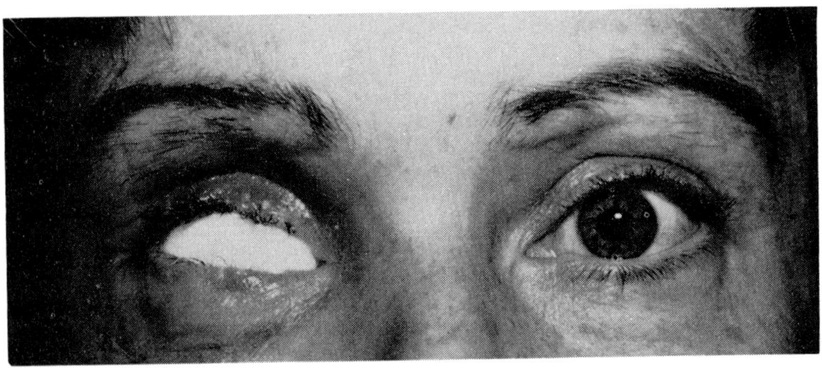

FIGURE 12.

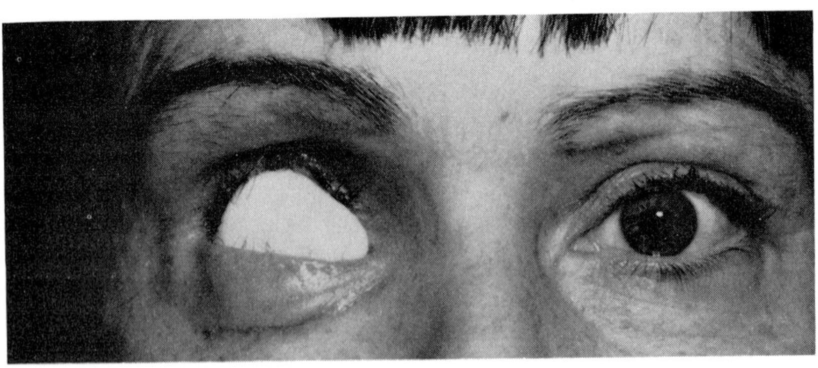

FIGURE 13.

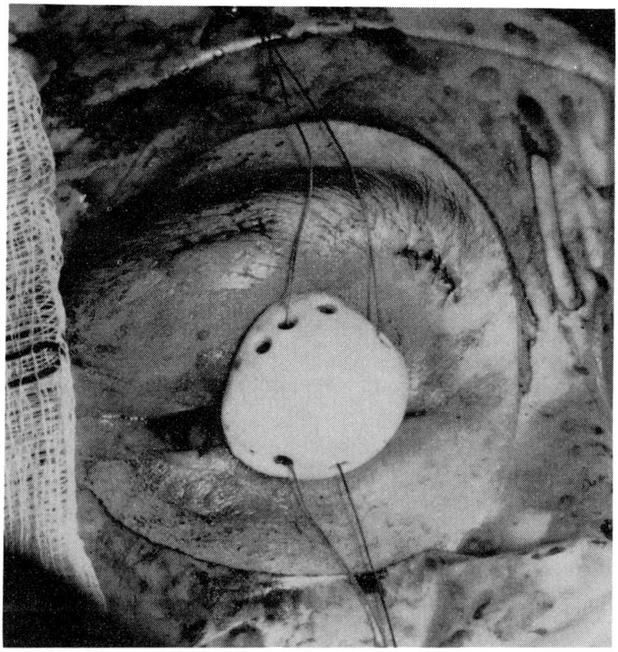

FIGURE 14.

taken from the mouth, over a large conformer should be inserted into the socket and left for as long as three to six months. The intrinsic fixation to the bone allows the patient to tolerate the procedure well for this period of time. Figure 15 shows the lower lid drawn down over the conformer and fastened to the cheek seven days after surgery. Despite this, scar tissue continued relentlessly and there was retraction primarily of the upper lid (Fig. 16) at the 14-week postoperative period. However, the conformer was extremely large and it was hoped that this would leave enough socket bed to accept a normal sized prosthesis.

When the wired or sutured conformer was removed at four months and a final prosthesis placed, the patient could close her lids readily over the prosthesis (Fig. 17). Eight months after surgery she had a most satisfactory cosmetic appearance with her prosthesis in place (Fig. 18), being able to wear one for the first time in five years. As pointed out by Callahan, it is essential that the patient maintain this prosthesis in place at all times because of the threat of socket contracture if removed for even a short period.

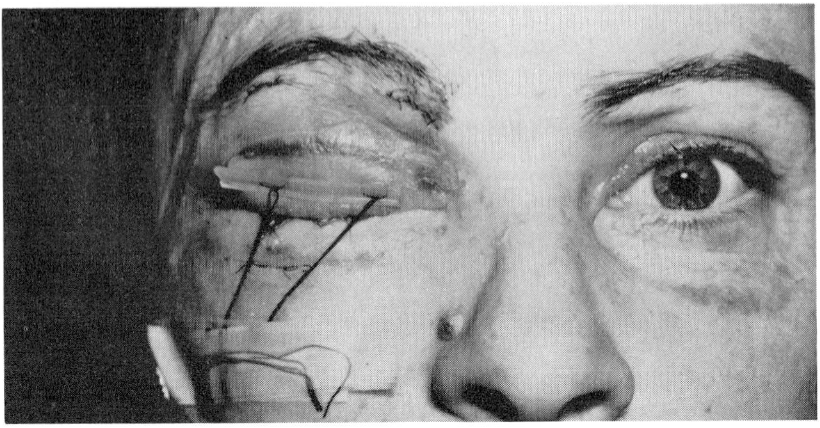

FIGURE 15.

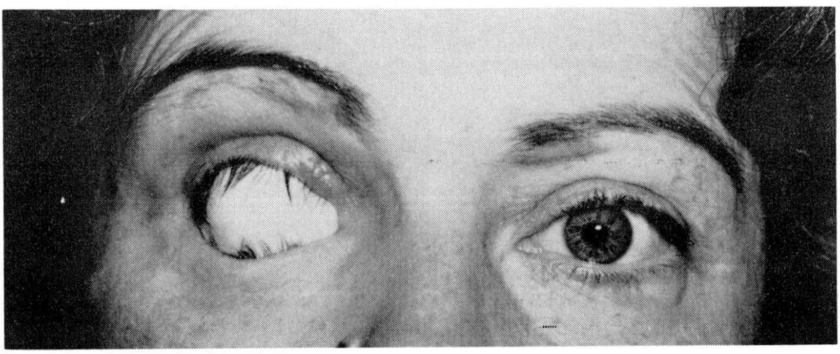

FIGURE 16.

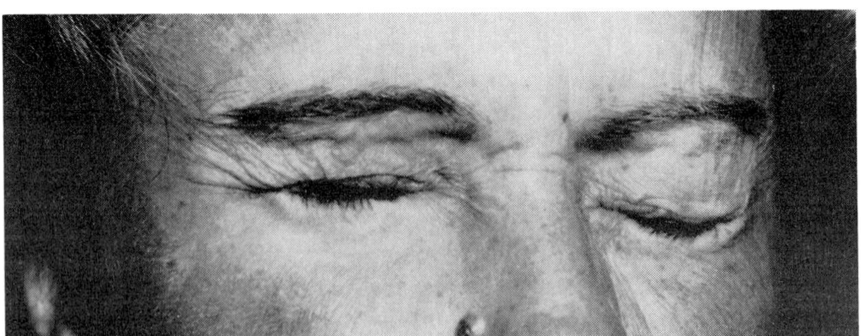

FIGURE 17.

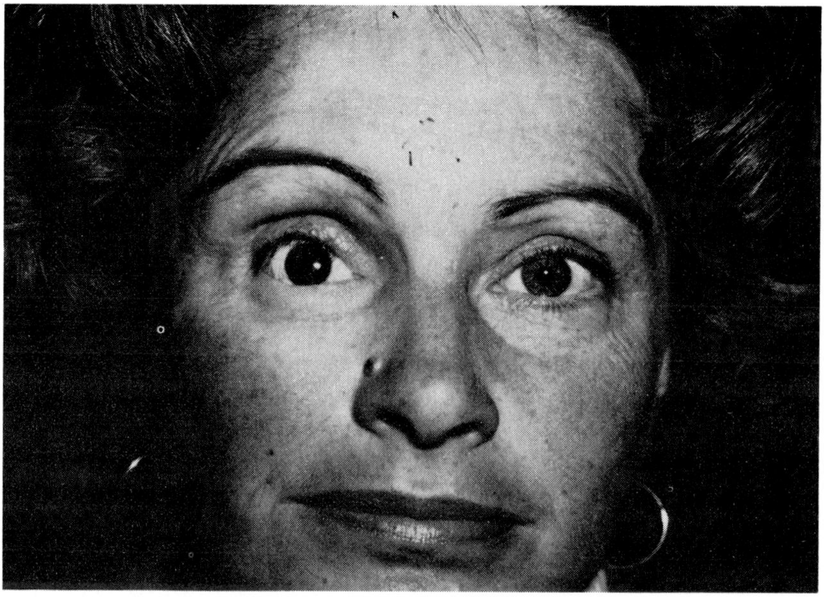

FIGURE 18.

The changes in an orbit should be carefully evaluated by x-ray study prior to surgery, and significant radical surgical procedures should be undertaken if one hopes to overcome the grossly contracted socket problem. In the presence of previous radiation, the x-ray evaluation is particularly significant, and it must be remembered that the vascularized scar tissues may be even more than the routine obstacle which one might otherwise encounter. "Think big" and aggressively for surgical reconstruction of the grossly contracted socket.

References

1. Small, R.: Influence of the ocularist and ophthalmologist in microorbit and microphthalmos. This volume.
2. Kennedy, R. E.: The effect of early enucleation on the orbit in animals and humans. Trans. Amer. Ophthal. Soc. 62:459, 1964; Amer. J. Ophthal. 60:277, 1965.
3. Kennedy, R. E.: Growth retardation and volume determinations of the anophthalmic orbit. Trans. Amer. Ophthal. Soc. 70:278, 1972; Amer. J. Ophthal. 76:294, 1973.
4. Callahan, A.: Symposium on surgery of the orbit and adnexa. *In* Transactions of the New Orleans Academy of Ophthalmology. St. Louis:The C. V. Mosby Co., 1974, p. 137.

III. Facial and Systemic

- Tumors
- Trauma
- Aging

Neurofibromatosis: Fitting Complications and Results

Robert A. Thomas

Socket reconstruction is a great challenge to ophthalmic surgeons:

> If someone attempts surgery early and there is a great deal of fibrous tissue the problem is ten times compounded. Once surgery is started in these sockets, it becomes a surgical problem over the years and the outlook is not nearly as favorable . . .
>
> Byron Smith, M.D.
> New York

The expansion of a fibrotic socket is a time-consuming procedure. A period of time, involving a number of conformer fittings, is required before the socket can retain a presentable prosthesis. However, the gratifying cosmetic appearance more than justifies the time and effort involved.

A 37-year-old man (Fig. 1A) was involved in an automobile accident in 1955. The damage to his left eye was so severe that it was necessary to enucleate the fragments. He was able to wear a prosthesis until 1972 when a growth appeared in the socket, pushing the prosthesis out. After removal of the growth, he came to the Eye Foundation Hospital. The examination showed the left socket was extremely contracted and socket reconstruction was attempted in December 1972 (Fig. 2). By March of 1973 the lid had receded behind the conformer and the lower fornix was completely lost. His ophthalmologist recommended that no further surgery be performed for at least a year, or possibly two, and referred him to us for a temporary solution. We inserted a series of "turnover" type conformers (Fig. 3). In two weeks, we noted the lower fornix had developed sufficiently to make it possible to obtain an impression of the socket. An impression-fitted champagne glass conformer was inserted. The pressure was maintained

Robert A. Thomas, Ocularist, The Eye Foundation Hospital, Birmingham, Ala.

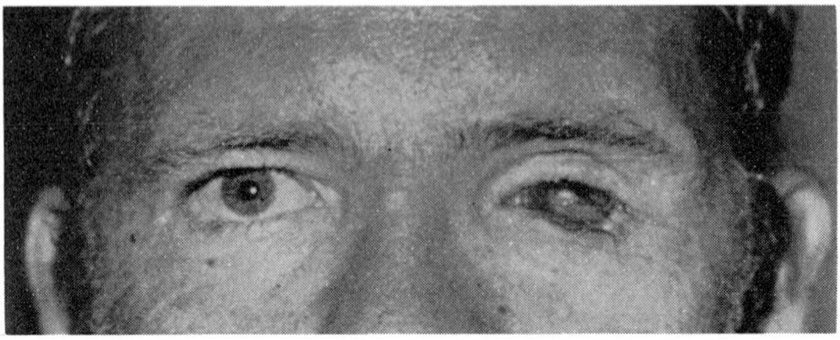

FIGURE 1.

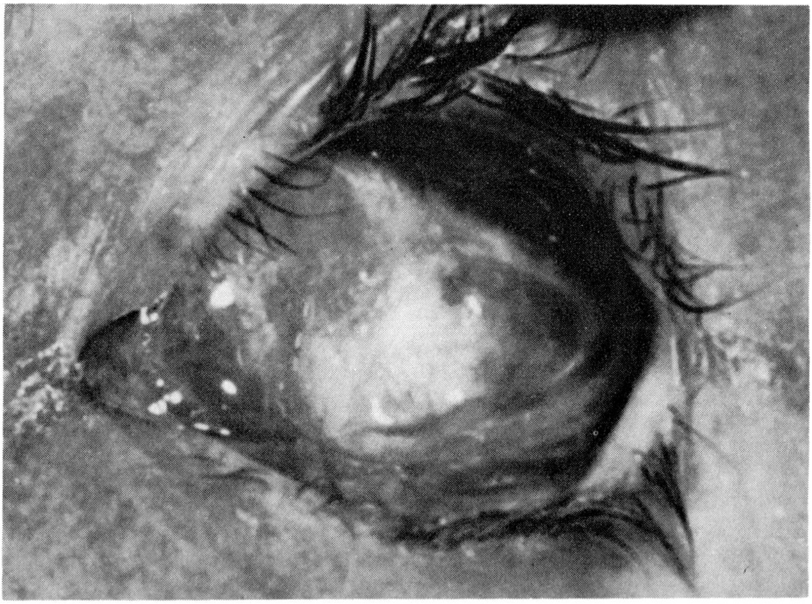

FIGURE 2.

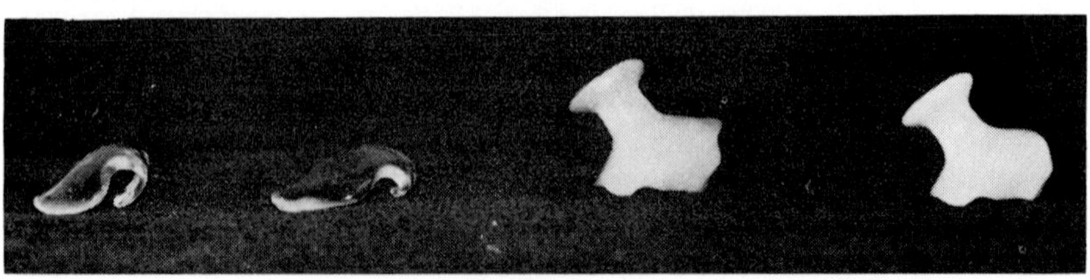

FIGURE 3.

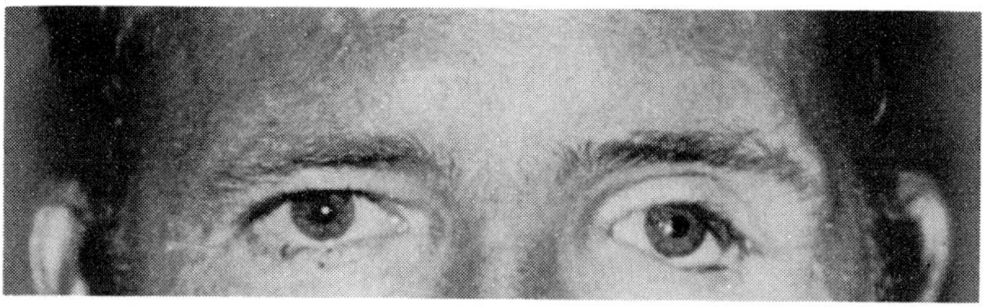

FIGURE 4.

with a bandage and tape. Four weeks later the custom-made prosthesis was inserted and retained (Fig. 4), and it has remained in place for 14 months.

A 59-year-old man had his left eye enucleated in 1950 as the result of an industrial accident. Numerous prosthetic eyes had been fitted prior to a socket reconstruction which was attempted in November 1973. Six weeks later the patient was unable to retain a prosthesis and upon examination presented a contracted fibrotic socket (Fig. 5). Over a nine-week period a series of three conformers (Fig. 6) was made to prepare his socket for the prosthesis, and held in place with the aid of a pressure bandage (Fig. 7). In February 1974 an impression for an ocular prosthesis was made. The impression showed the socket had assumed the shape of the "turnover" conformer. This technique resulted in an acceptable cosmetic effect (Fig. 8) and prompted the patient to comment, "I didn't believe it would stay in and I don't even feel it." Note that pressure was used in both of these fibrotic socket expansion cases.

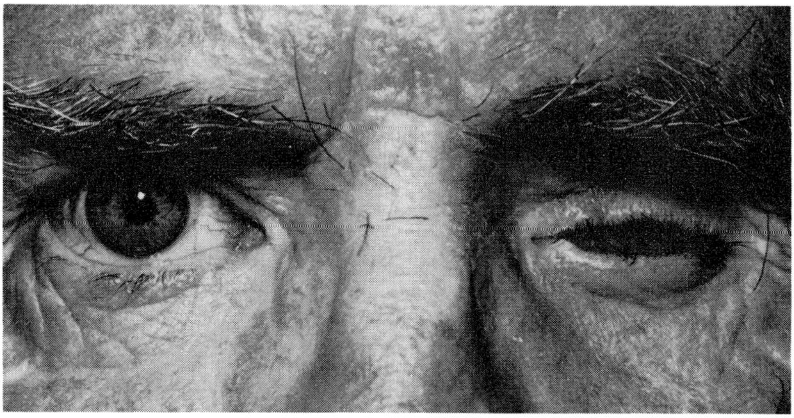

FIGURE 5.

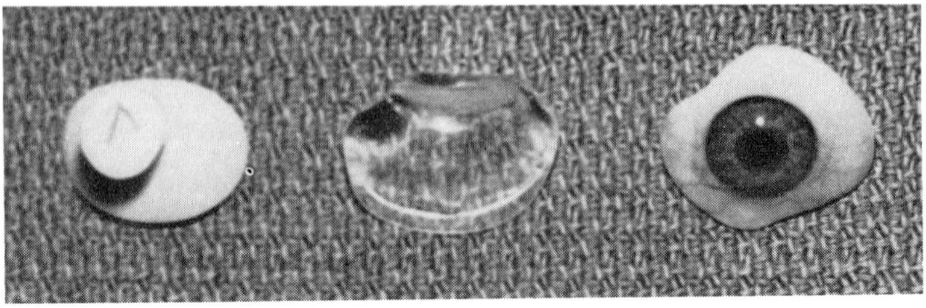

FIGURE 6.

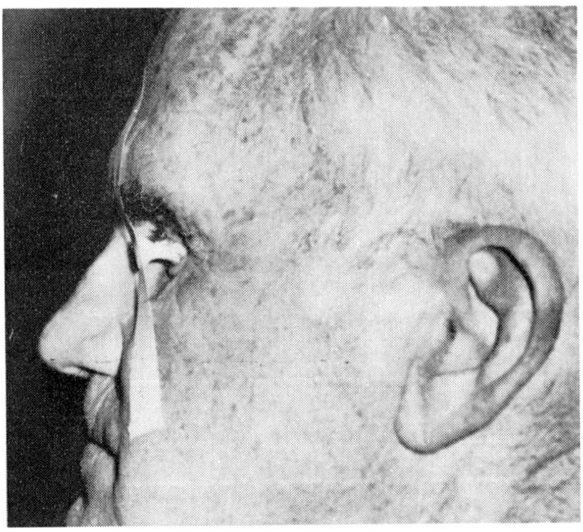

FIGURE 7.

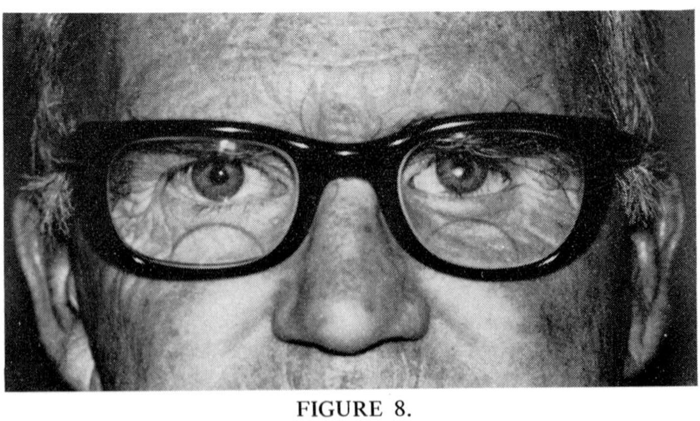

FIGURE 8.

A man, 29 years of age, had lost his right eye as the result of an automobile accident in December 1972. Examination showed upper and lower lid-margin lacerations with formation of scar tissue and symblepharon from medial canthus to upper lid and multiple facial fractures (Fig. 9). In May 1973 a major socket reconstruction was performed using a buccal mucosal graft. A stock eye which had tunnels drilled through the anterior surface (Fig. 10) was used as a conformer and was sutured into place. The sutures were passed through the lids and tied in place over cotton pledgets (Fig. 11). In November the prosthetic conformer was removed (Fig. 12) and an impression procedure for an ocular prosthesis was carried out. Periodic checkups and adjustments have been made to the prosthesis over the past ten months in an effort to achieve the best possible cosmetic effect (Fig. 13).

A 22-year-old man suffered caustic burns to both eyes in May 1973. The right eye was eviscerated (Fig. 14), leaving a completely scarred corneal surface with symblepharon (Fig. 15). Surgery was performed at the Eye Foundation Hospital in May 1974 for socket reconstruction with mucosal grafts. In July a cosmetic, therapeutic,

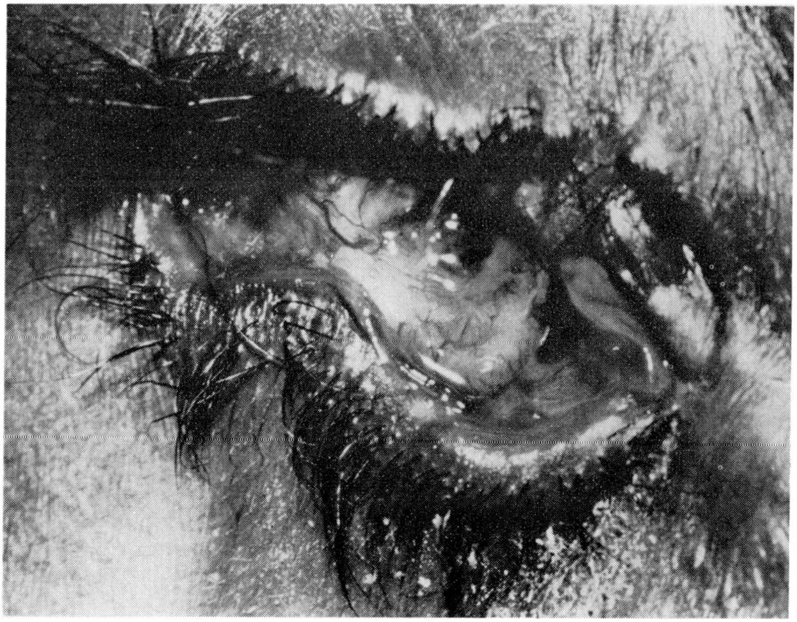

FIGURE 9.

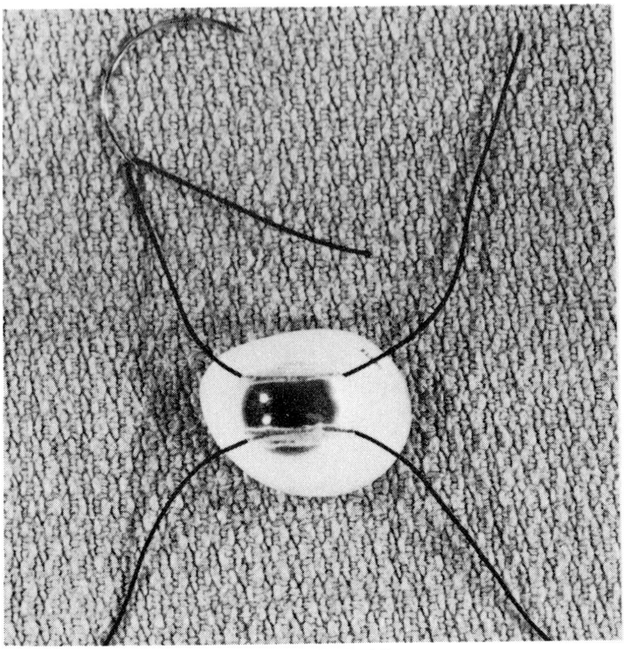

FIGURE 10.

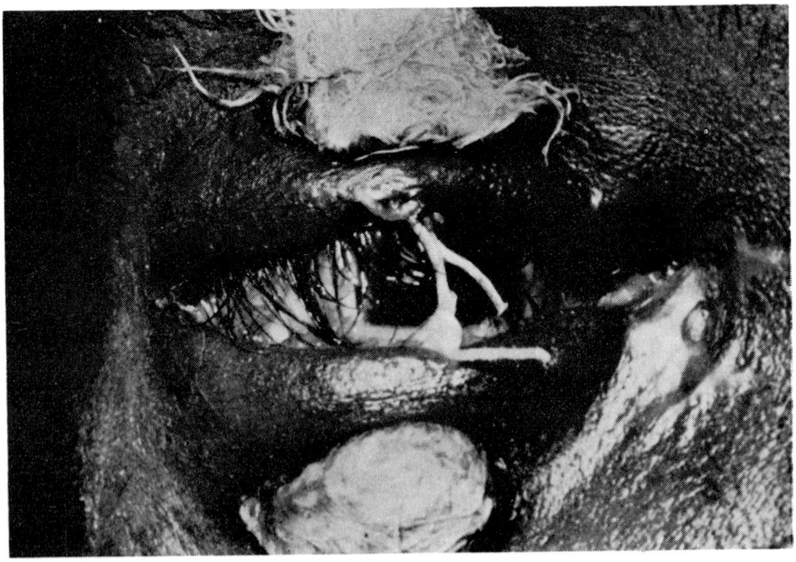

FIGURE 11.

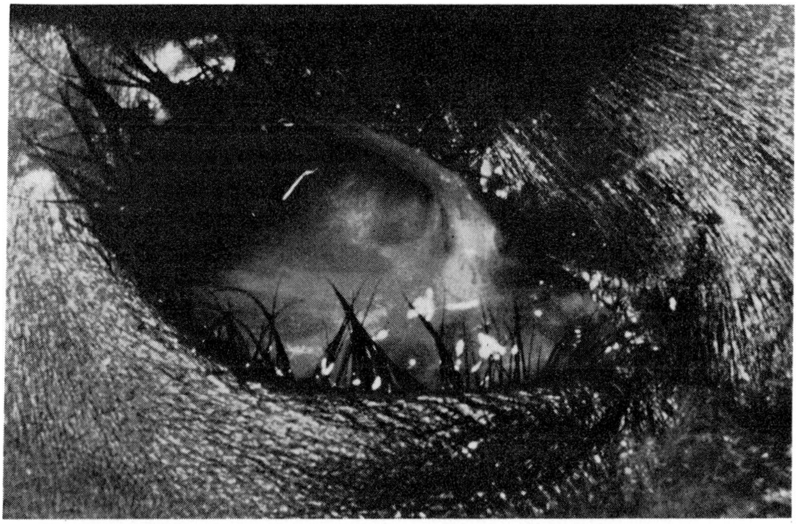

FIGURE 12.

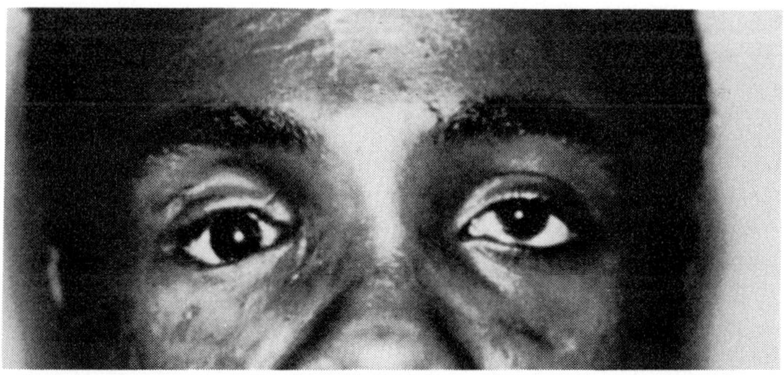

FIGURE 13.

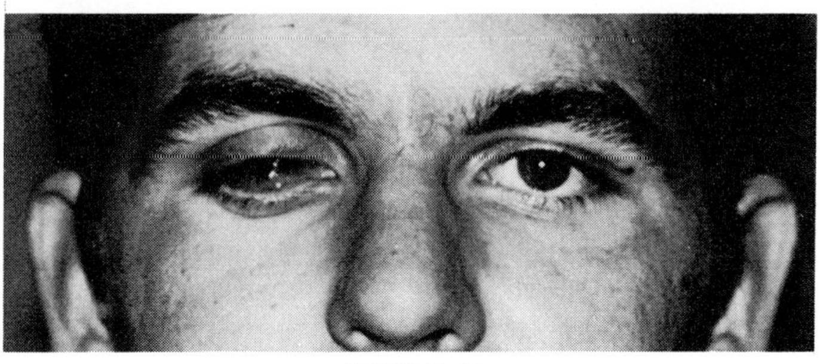

FIGURE 14.

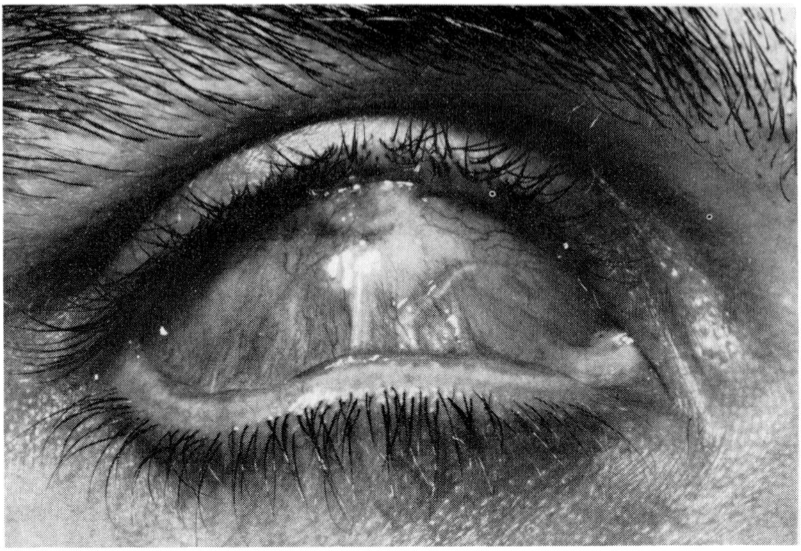

FIGURE 15.

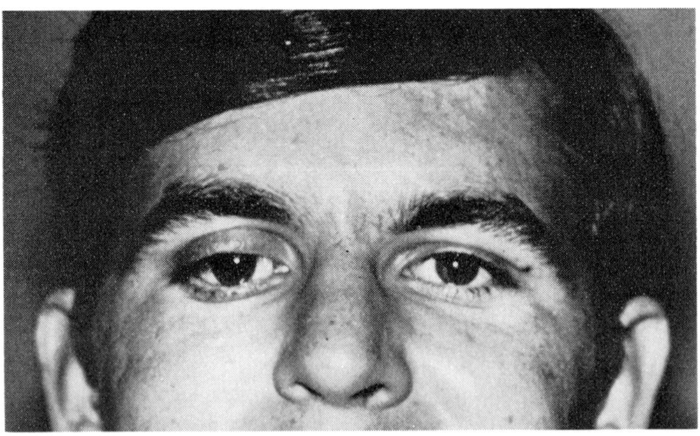

FIGURE 16.

shell was fabricated. The patient was able to tolerate it comfortably until August. The shell was cracked during cleaning and a new shell was fabricated, at which time we noted the upper and lower fornices had further developed. The prosthesis was altered to improve cosmetic effect (Fig. 16).

Summary

It has been the assumption that only congenital anophthalmic sockets could be expanded with the use of conformers of increasing size. We have attempted expansion in five cases and have had gratifying results. The ocularist has a number of procedures available for dealing with a fibrotic socket. These innovative procedures are the result of a close partnership between the ophthalmologist and ocularist. If we are to continue improving our patient services, we must expand this partnership.

Anophthalmos and Neurofibromatosis

David B. Soll, M.D.

The number of patients with neurofibromatosis who have an anophthalmic socket is quite small. Enucleation may become necessary when the globe becomes extremely proptotic, uncontrollable glaucoma is present, or optic nerve tumors occur.

Some authorities differentiate between the multiple, plexiform type of neurofibroma as compared with the solitary orbital form. The former may be accompanied by elephantiasis neuromatosa, which is a pendulous hypertrophy and thickening of the upper eyelid skin, and is not amenable to full surgical excision; whereas the solitary tumor, usually presenting in an older age group, may be removed and, as a rule, does not recur.

In dealing with the plexiform type, the globe may have to be enucleated. In any anophthalmic socket, I generally prefer the use of a fascia lata sling technique for correcting the ptosis. Autogenous fascia lata is preferred since it is more permanent, whereas donor fascia lata tends to absorb. The S-shaped deformity, so frequently present, also may be improved with the use of selectively placed fascia lata slings.

In certain instances it is possible to excise the involved section of the levator muscle and upper eyelid tissue, thus horizontally shortening a lax upper eyelid. This may be combined with a levator muscle resection.

The problem of an anophthalmic socket associated with neurofibromatosis of the orbit is a challenging one and each case must be considered individually.

David B. Soll, M.D., F.A.C.S., Professor and Chairman, Department of Ophthalmology, Hahnemann Medical College and Hospital, Philadelphia; Director, Department of Ophthalmology, Rolling Hill Hospital, Elkins Park, and Frankford Hospital, Philadelphia, Pa.

Use of Prosthetics to Camouflage Facial, Lid and Ocular Deformities

Clarence W. Cox, Jr.

In these modern times, patients are usually referred to ocularists for artificial eyes. Our skills in working with acrylics and similar materials, our gratification in helping physicians restore normal appearances to the patients and sometimes the proximity of our laboratories make it natural that we would receive referrals for special-purpose prosthetic devices.

The first device to be presented is the ptosis crutch (Fig. 1). There has always been a need for this, but in the past those available either did not hold the lid securely or pressed too tightly. It is used to elevate the upper lid when muscle or nerve function has been lost. We have developed a ptosis crutch which allows the patient to blink his eye, and it may be worn during all the waking hours. With the old, rigid ptosis crutches this was not possible.

A 58-year-old man was referred to the prosthetic department for help with traumatic ptosis of the right upper lid. It was thought by the physician that the condition might be temporary, so a solution other than surgery was considered to be the best approach. A 22-gauge stainless steel spring wire was utilized to make a flexible ptosis crutch. The wire was bent into two loops to allow fixation with two small screws to the spectacle frame. A right-angle bend was made above the two loops and a three-loop coil spring was wound into the wire. Another right-angle bend was made in the wire which allowed it to extend across the lid, and it was curved to fit into the lid fold. This was then covered with a piece of polyethylene tubing from a scalp vein needle set. It worked quite well. The patient was able to completely close his eye (Fig. 2A), the ptosis crutch opened his eye fully (Fig. 2B), the palpebral fissure was reasonably shaped, and the crutch was not visible. After eight months it became obvious that this was a permanent disability, and his levator muscle was resected to permanently correct his ptosis.

Clarence W. Cox, Jr., Ocularist, The Eye Foundation Hospital, Birmingham, Ala.

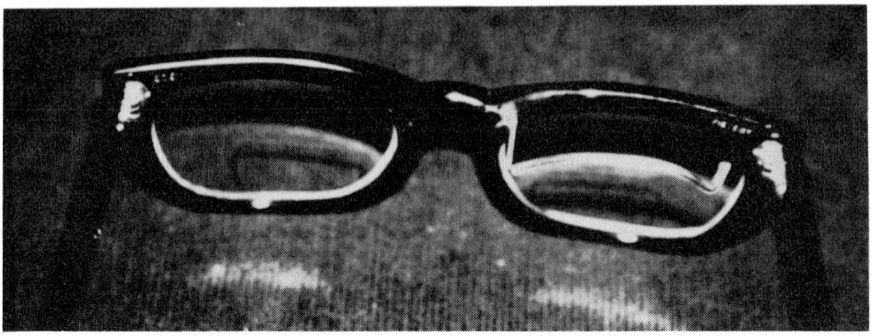

FIG. 1. Ptosis crutch.

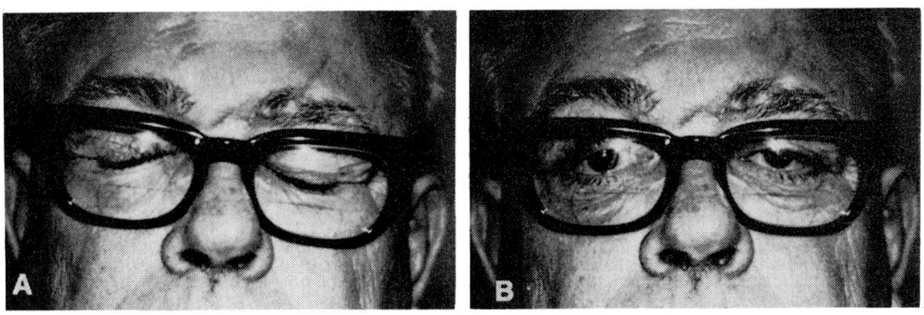

FIG. 2. (A) Patient left with paralyzed eyelid after trauma. The ptosis crutch allows him to close his eye. (B) The ptosis crutch effectively and fully opens his eye.

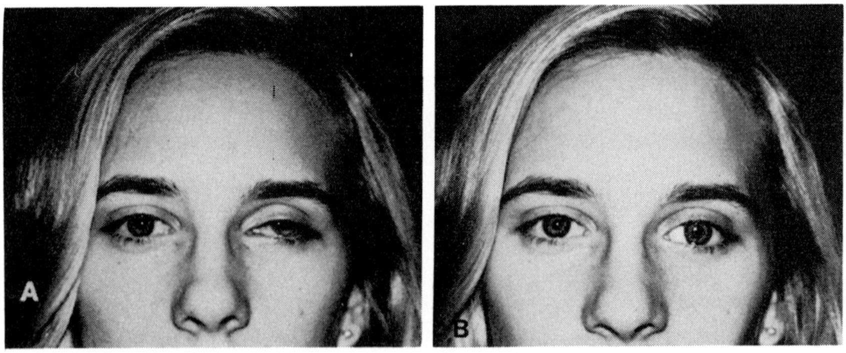

FIG. 3. (A) A 16-year-old girl with an evisceration and Silastic ball implant following glaucoma. (B) Satisfactory result after being fitted with a cosmetic shell.

A 16-year-old girl who had an evisceration with a Silastic ball implant after a history of glaucoma (Fig. 3A) was fitted with a cosmetic shell with a satisfactory result (Fig. 3B).

A 58-year-old woman was referred to us because her prosthetic eye was improperly shaped and had pushed the lower lid down, causing a rounding and drooping of the palpebral fissure (Fig. 4A). The socket was barely retaining her artificial eye. On examination we found that the patient had been fitted with a Snellen reform eye (Fig. 4B), which had been placed over a well-secured Allen implant. The patient was refitted, using the modified impression method. Unfortunately she had worn the ill-fitting eye so long that it was not possible to fit the socket perfectly, but we did improve the appearance and, even more important, we prevented further erosion of the conjunctiva and the Tenon's capsule over

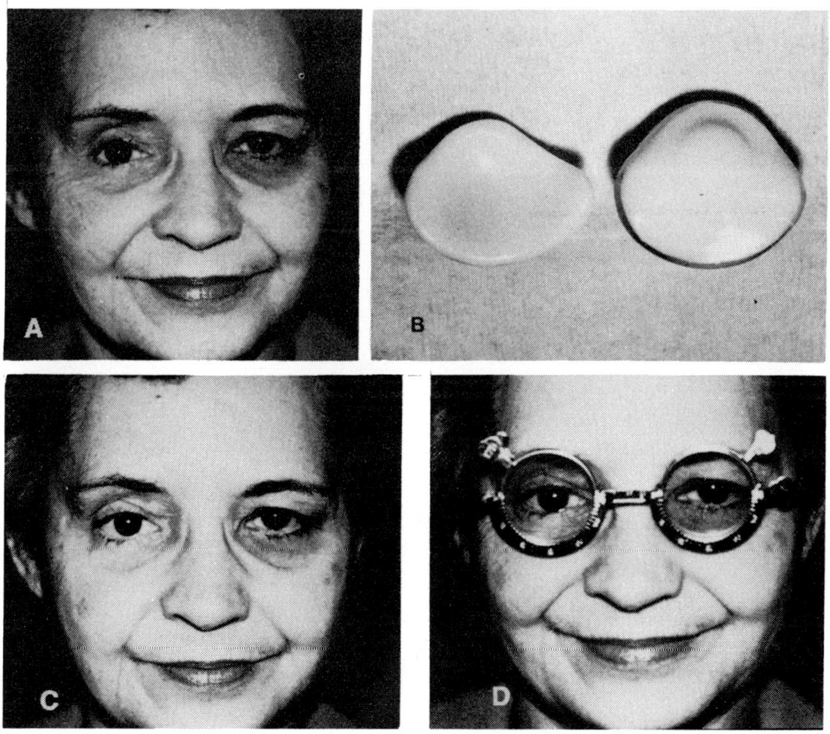

FIG. 4. (A) Patient whose ill-fitting artificial eye caused rounding and drooping of the palpebral fissure. (B) Comparison of Snellen reform (left) and impression-fitted (right) artificial eyes. (C) The patient wearing the impression-fitted prosthetic eye. (D) Cosmetic optics used in the final correction.

the implant (Fig. 4C). For the final correction we used cosmetic optics (Fig. 4D). We have found that very good results may be obtained by using the full-size trial lens set and placing the patient's prescription over the good eye. We can then compare the appearance of the natural eye with the prosthetic eye.

Sometimes it is possible to achieve the desired result with a very simple approach. A young man was referred to us who had lost the central portion of his upper left lid margin in an automobile accident. A subsequent surgical reconstruction allowed the socket to retain an impression-fitted prosthesis, but the lack of an upper lid margin detracted from the overall appearance (Fig. 5A). An artificial eyelash was attached to the lid fold centrally and to the lid margin on the medial and lateral aspects (Fig. 5B). This effectively masked the defect, and the patient is very happy with it and does not object to wearing an artificial eyelash.

A 53-year-old man was seen in the clinic at the Eye Foundation Hospital (Fig. 6A). It was noted that the patient had received severe

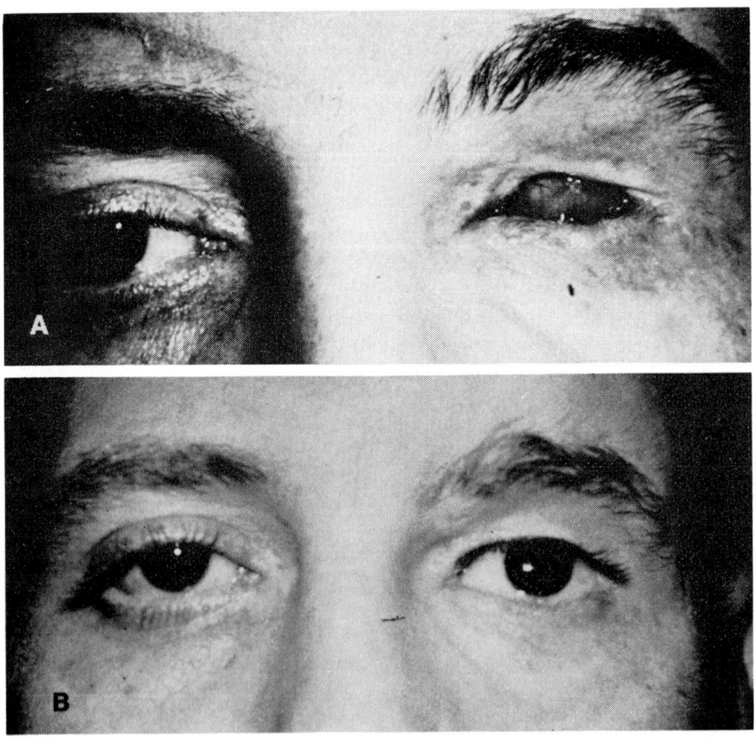

FIG. 5. (A) Patient with loss of the medial section of his upper eyelid. (B) The defect masked by an artificial eyelash.

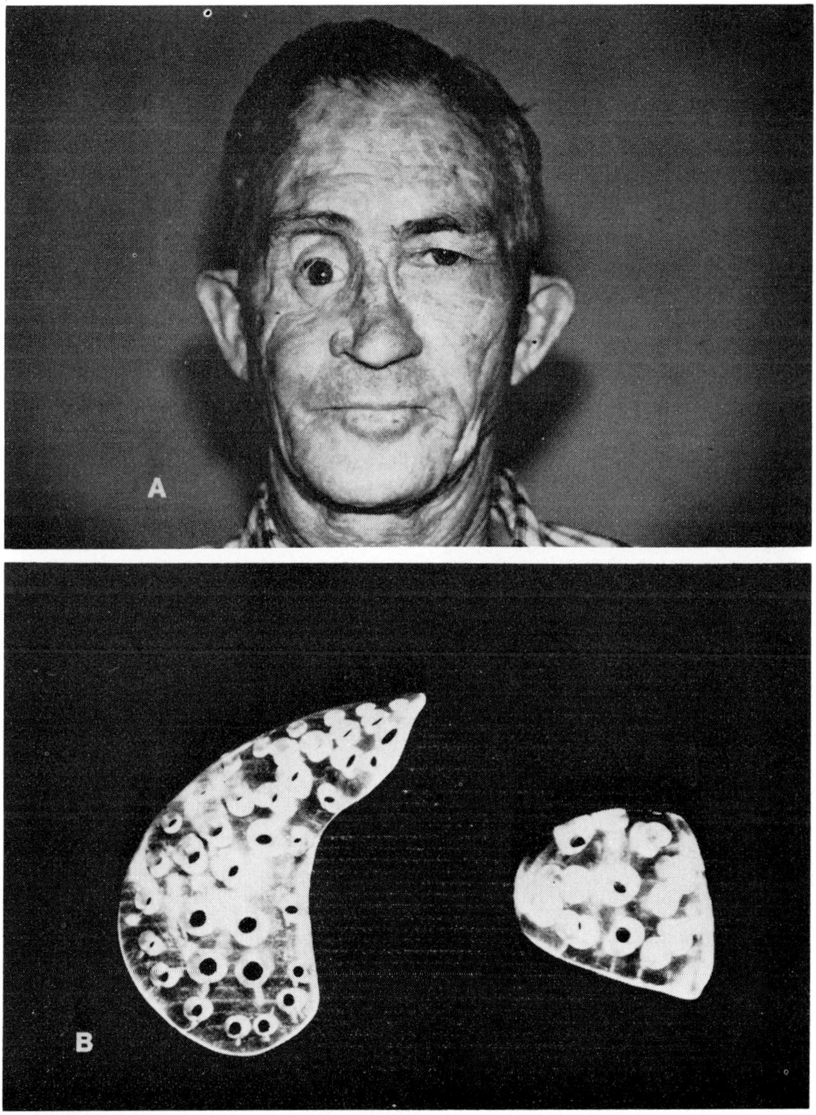

FIG. 6. (A) A 53-year-old man with multiple facial and orbital defects. (B) Custom-made implants fabricated for the patient. (C) Implants carried out in both acrylic and Silastic. (D) Clear "turnover" conformer used to reestablish the inferior fornix. (E) Result improved by using cosmetic optics in his spectacles.

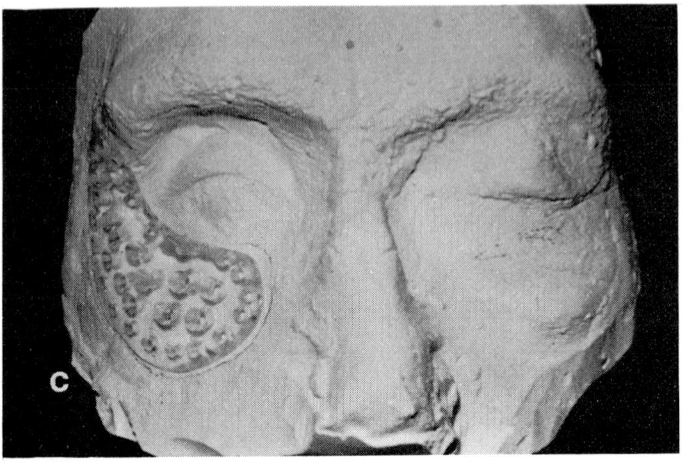

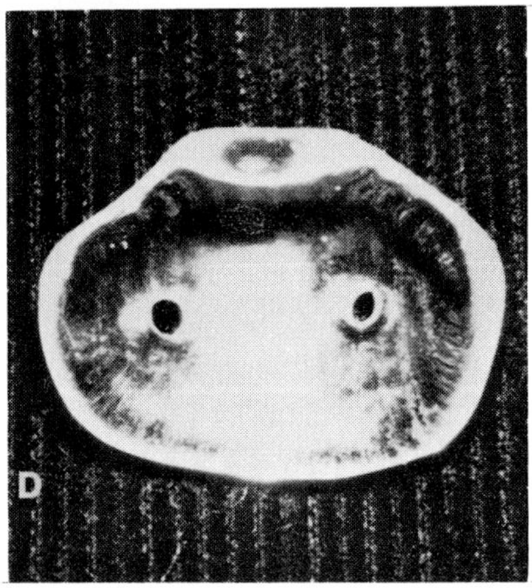

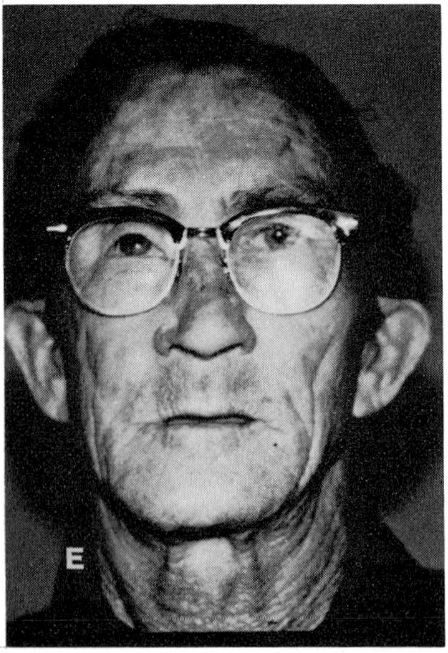

FIG. 6. (Continued)

damage to the lateral and the infraorbital rims. It was possible for the socket to retain an artificial eye, but the result was poor due to the extremely deep sulcus, loss of the lateral and infraorbital rims and a 1-cm inferior displacement of the socket. On consultation with the resident assigned to the case and the attending physician, it was decided that custom-made implants should be fabricated for this patient (Fig. 6B). This was carried out in both acrylic and Silastic (Fig. 6C). The Silastic implants were chosen at the time of surgery. The implant for the floor of the orbit was made in the shape of the end of the thumb with the end turned up, to push the contents of the orbit up to fill the sulcus. A standard conformer was placed in the socket. The patient lost the conformer after a few days but did not report this to the physician or the ocularist, resulting in the loss of the lower fornix. A clear "turnover" type conformer was used to reestablish the left inferior fornix (Fig. 6D). After the patient had worn the turnover conformer for about a month an artificial eye was fabricated for him (Fig. 6E). The result was improved somewhat by using the prescription in his right lens of plano +4.0 diopters at 130° with 4° base down prism and a 2.5 diopter add. This created the illusion of raising the orbit, which was still inferiorly displaced after his plastic surgery and artificial eye were completed.

A 9-year-old girl was referred to us by a physician who had done a complete exenteration for a rhabdomyosarcoma (Fig. 7A). The physician reported that the malignancy was arrested and asked us to help this lovely young girl. It was decided that an external orbital prosthesis should be fabricated and attached to the glasses (Fig. 7B). Recently she had another small graft operation due to the failure of the orbit to heal in the back. A biopsy was found not to be malignant. The prosthesis still fits.

In patients in whom there is complete obliteration of the orbit, the obvious best help is an external orbital prosthesis. In some cases there is a question as to the best approach, and the patient should be informed as to what may be expected from surgery and what can be done with a prosthesis, and then allowed to make a decision. The 28-year-old woman shown in Figure 8A lost her left eye at age 2 as a result of retinoblastoma. Radiation was used at that time and the tissues had contracted over the years until it was impossible for her to wear an artificial eye. She refused to have surgery but wholeheartedly accepted the external orbital prosthesis and wears it proudly (Fig. 8B).

In summary, we are sometimes surprised at how simple a thing can alleviate a problem which has caused a patient much grief and heartache.

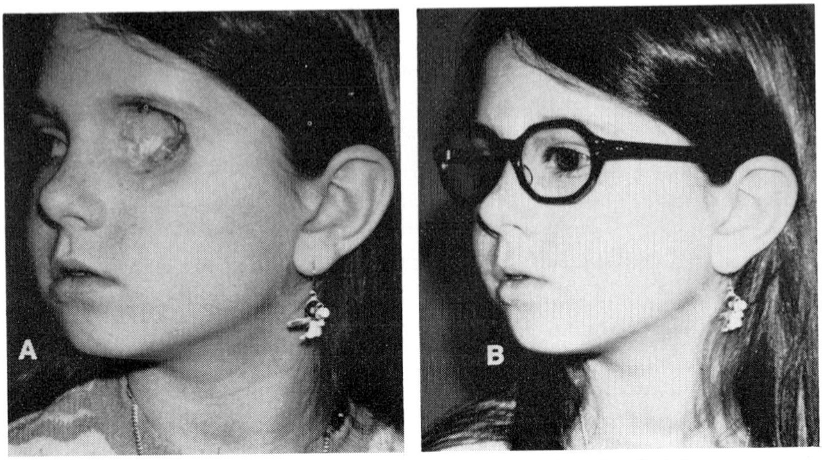

FIG. 7. (A) A 9-year-old girl with a complete exenteration for rhabdomyosarcoma. (B) External orbital prosthesis in place.

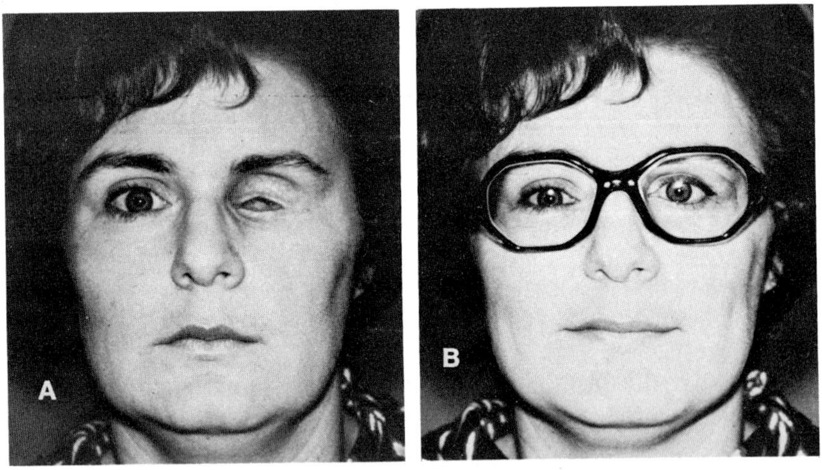

FIG. 8. (A) A 28-year-old woman with a severely contracted socket caused by the use of radiation. (B) Improved appearance with an external orbital prosthesis.

We must keep in mind that patients with ocular and facial deformities caused by trauma or disease have a very real psychological problem, and anything that we can contribute toward allaying their fears and anxieties will be well worth the time and trouble it takes.

Repair and Camouflage of Orbital and Ocular Deformities

Allison J. Berlin, Jr., M.D.

Of the many disabilities or handicaps which can afflict man, facial disfigurement is one of tragic proportions [1]. It is a misfortune compounded by a special irony in that it is rarely disabling physically. The patient's reaction to his physical asymmetry is a realistic response to a socially observed fact. This adversity stems from the almost obsessive concern with physical attributes in our highly competitive society. Incredibly, the disability usually does not restict one's ability to work or perform his normal daily activities and yet remains an extreme handicap with great social and psychological ramifications. So it is that we, by choice, spend significant amounts of time in dealing with the problems associated with such facial and orbital disfigurement.

There are a multiplicity of techniques available in the repair and camouflage of orbital and ocular deformities. Since an extensive review of such procedures is not feasible, I have chosen a few techniques which have been helpful in this area.

Eyelid deformities from trauma are due to scar contracture, malposition or distortion of the tissues through faulty suturing of a laceration, and varying amounts of tissue destruction or contractures resulting from burns. Converse notes that such deformities may involve the skin alone, the lid margin or a part of the full thickness or entire full thickness of the lid [2]. Deformity from contracture is usually caused by vertical scars which pull the lid out of the normal alignment and may cause notching of the free margin. If possible, simple excision of the scars and accurate anatomic anastomosis of the lid margins will be sufficient to restore good anatomic contour (Fig. 1). If cicatricial retraction occurs with notching of the eyelid margin, it may be necessary to avoid the straight-line suture.

Allison J. Berlin, Jr., M.D., Department of Ophthalmology, The Cleveland Clinic, Cleveland, Ohio.

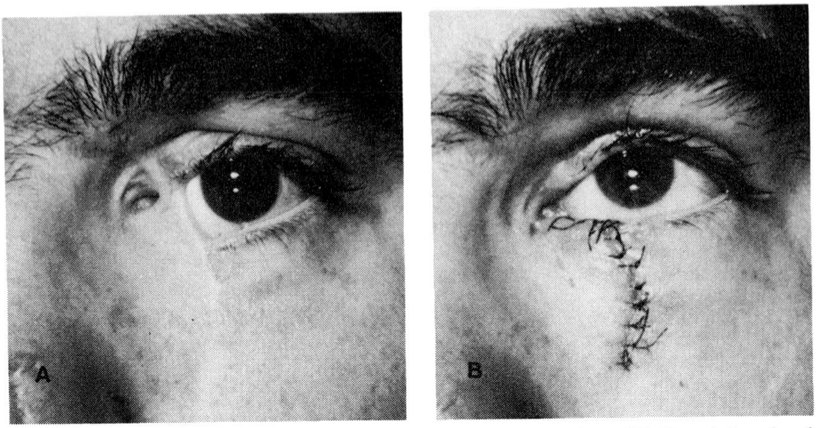

FIG. 1. (A) Faulty primary closure of extensive lid laceration. (B) Repair by simple excision of scar and realignment of lid margins.

The Z-plasty technique breaks up the straight-line scar and, in addition, elongates the vertical dimension of the lid involved (Fig. 2).

If antitension-line techniques are not sufficient to give adequate relaxation of the contracted lid, it may be necessary to apply a full-thickness or split-thickness skin graft to the contracted area. Full-thickness skin grafts should be taken in order of preference from the lid or orbital area, followed by the retroauricular area. Split-thickness skin grafts, if necessary, may be taken from the area closest to the face to give the best color match.

Facial burns frequently produce more extensive and severe ectropion. The treatment of burn ectropion involves the primary use of split-thickness skin grafts employed in the upper eyelids to reproduce the thin skin of the upper eyelid. Full-thickness retroauricular or supraclavicular grafts are employed in ectropion of the lower eyelid skin. The thick graft generally works more satisfactorily in the less mobile lower lid.

Chemical burns, usually of the alkali type, produce orbital contraction in addition to loss of the globe. Reconstruction of the fornices of the orbit by means of mucous membrane grafts and subsequent recontouring of the orbital prosthesis may be helpful in reducing the deformity. Most socket contractures from alkali burns are extremely difficult problems and may continue to contract for years after the original injury.

The patient shown in Figure 3 suffered an alkali burn to his orbit and loss of the eye some 12 years earlier. He had continuous contraction of his lower lid over the years with multiple surgical procedures. Analysis of the

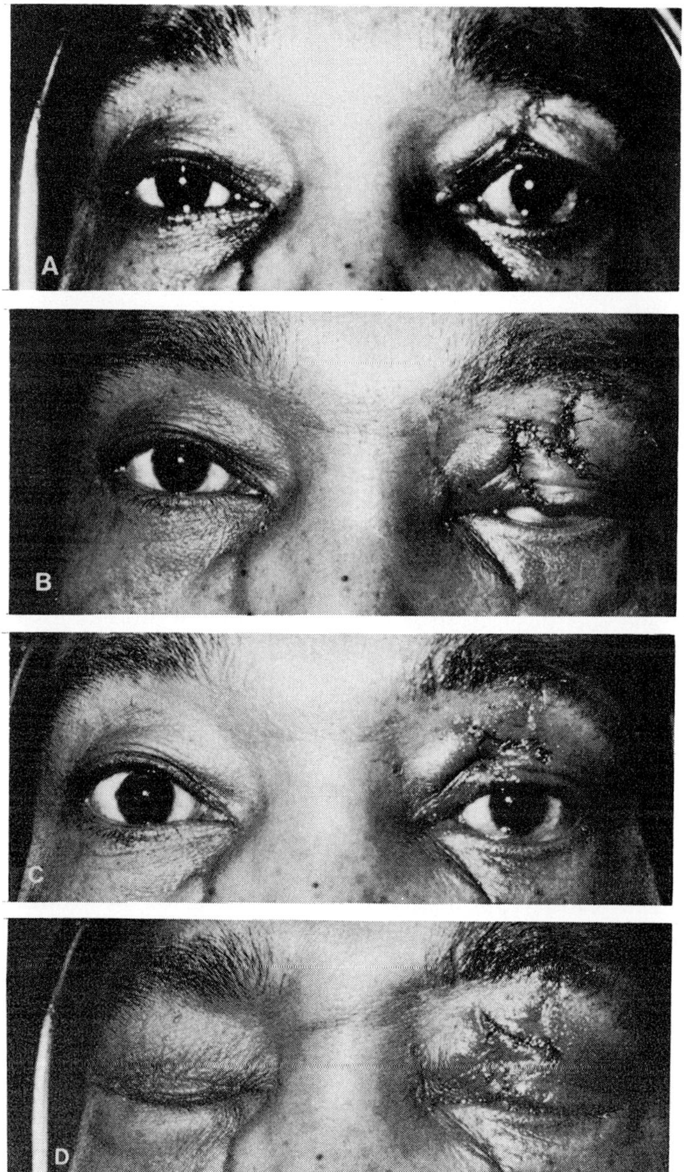

FIG. 2. (A and B) Straight-line scar of left upper lid after trauma with retraction. (C and D) Elimination of retraction by Z-plasty technique.

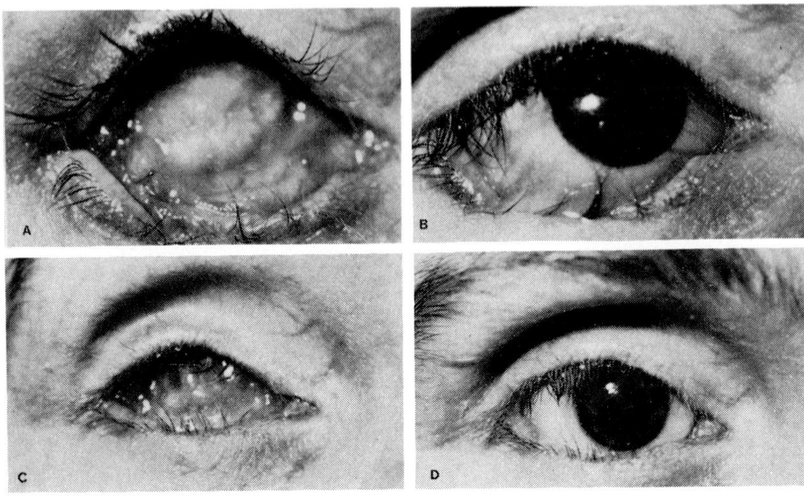

FIG. 3. (A and B) Alkali burn to right orbit with inability to retain prosthesis. (C and D) Reconstruction of lower lid using nasal mucous membrane graft.

defect revealed a contracture of the lower lid with granulation tissue in the socket and the lower lid from his previous surgical procedures. Mustarde has proposed the use of nasal mucosa as a support in the reconstruction of the lower lid defects after removal for neoplasms [2]. Borrowing his suggestion in terms of resisting lid contraction, a nasal mucous membrane graft was inserted in the patient's lower lid with satisfactory correction of the deformity and subsequent retention of his ocular prosthesis.

Lid and ocular deformities may pose a problem for both the ophthalmic plastic surgeon and the ocularist. Scar revision may be performed to eliminate the cosmetic lid deformity. Z-plasty or mucous membrane grafting will eliminate the symblepharon or shortening and contraction of the fornices, and permit the fitting of a cosmetic shell.

The woman shown in Figure 4 presented with remote trauma following an auto injury. She was extremely concerned about her appearance and wished cosmetic improvement in this left orbit. Examination revealed displacement of the lid structures as well as symblepharon to the blind phthisical eye. A revision of her scar with resuturing of the lid margins produced improvement in the anatomic appearance of the lid. A Z-plasty to the conjunctiva relieved the symblepharon and allowed sufficient space for the insertion of a cosmetic shell.

The ocularist has been particularly helpful in devising scleral shells which very closely mimic the appearance of a normal eye in camouflaging

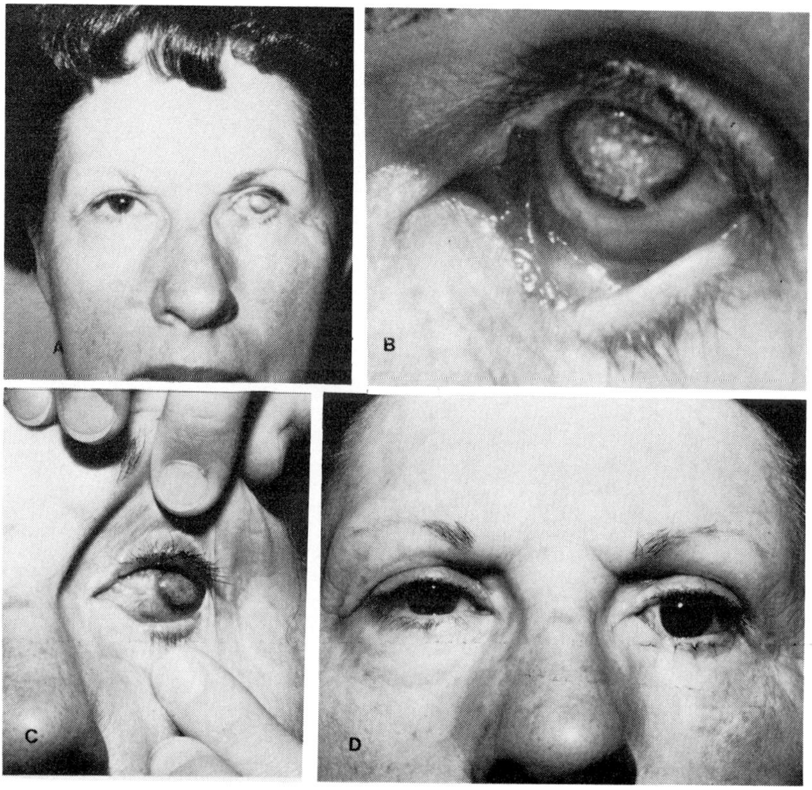

FIG. 4. (A and B) Trauma to the left orbit with notching of the lid and symblepharon. (C and D) After revision of the lid scar and Z-plasty to the conjunctiva, a cosmetic shell could be worn.

the phthisical shrunken globe or the eviscerated shell. Good motility may be elicited in these cases with satisfactory camouflage of the deformity.

Orbital rim fractures often result in bone depression. A number of techniques have been utilized to manage this type of problem. Overlay bone grafts, bone chips, Cranioplast and silicone have all been employed. (I am particularly indebted to the Department of Plastic Surgery at the Cleveland Clinic for their thinking and original contributions in this area.) Bone deformity of the rim with depression has been approached by reconstituting the rim with a silicone prosthesis (Fig. 5). This technique utilizes a fast-setting gel-like substance called Super Gel for making a mask of the face and thus the orbital deformity. The Super Gel is mixed and molded over the patient's face with straws inserted in the nostrils to allow

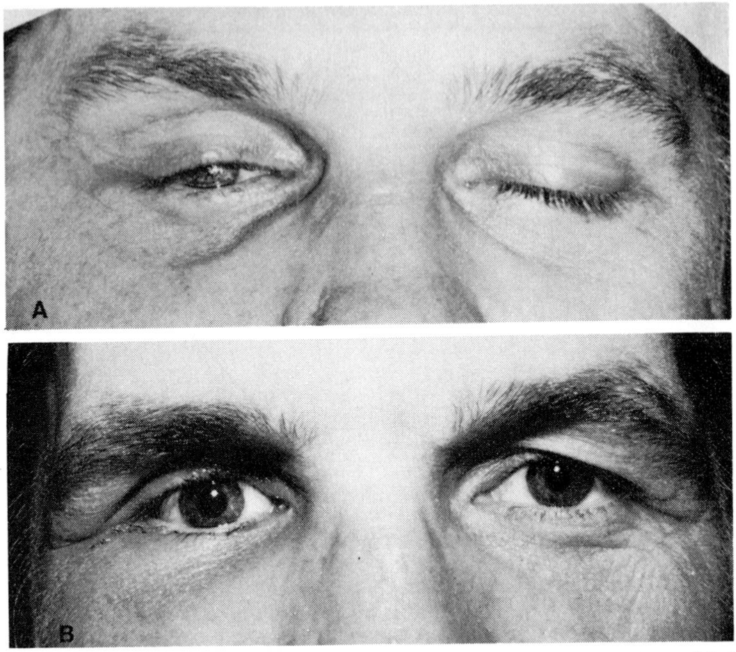

FIG. 5. (A) Traumatic fracture to the right orbit with severe depression of inferior orbital rim. (B) Postoperative view immediately after insertion of silicone prosthesis.

the patient to breathe while the gel is setting. When the gel is peeled off the face, a negative cast of the face is produced. Into this negative cast, impression plaster is poured to produce a positive mold of the face. The deformity of the orbital rim is then filled utilizing dental wax. From this malleable type of mold, a Silastic implant is shaped by hand. Surgically, a lower lid incision is made with dissection anterior to the orbicularis down to the orbital rim, at which point the periosteum is incised and elevated to create a pocket between the periosteum and anterior facial bones. The silicone prosthesis is inserted into this pocket with reshaping as necessary. The periosteum is closed to the deep orbital tissues at the top of the pocket.

In summary, many techniques are available for the management of orbital and ocular deformities. Some of these are applicable with or without the globe. Others are specifically designed to handle the problem of the anophthalmic socket. All are designed to aid the patient in reducing his anxiety and the social stigma from his orbital trauma.

References

1. Kazanjian, V. H. and Converse, J. M.: Surgical Treatment of Facial Injuries, 3rd ed. Baltimore: Williams & Wilkins Co., 1974, pp. 440, 630.
2. Mustarde, J. C.: Repair and Reconstruction in the Orbital Region. Baltimore: Williams & Wilkins Co., 1966.

Prosthetic Considerations in the Aging Patient

Marsha Erickson Guibor, C.O.

The prosthetic considerations in the aging patient include blepharosulcus depression often complicated by blepharoptosis and a sagging lower lid. Blepharosulcus depression may not always be considered a deformity per se if the condition is bilateral (Fig. 1). However, when blepharosulcus depression exists unilaterally, it is an unsightly deformity that requires surgical or nonsurgical correction (Fig. 2). *Surgical correction* may be considered in three aspects: subperiosteal implantation, implantation inferior to the supraorbital rim or cosmetic blepharoplasty of the upper lid of the alternate eye. *Nonsurgical correction* may best be attempted with an impression-fitted prosthesis.

Impressions of the socket may be taken with impression shells or trays as shown in Figure 3; however, they are often unsatisfactory in that they are too large or too small, thus yielding an impression which has to be modified so extensively to fulfill such an elementary criterion as a matching palpebral fissure that the final prosthesis may not resemble the initial impression.

There has been substantial controversy regarding whether an impression- or nonimpression-type prosthesis yields the highest motility and whether the motility is derived from the fornices or from the shape and movement of the tissues and implant. The following technique is a combination of the two techniques (impression and nonimpression) and therefore may take best advantage of the merits of both theories.

A custom-made, empirically fitted, wax molding shell or tray is created. It may be held with a suction cup (Fig. 4) for the insertion technique (the impression material is placed on the posterior side of the molding shell and then *inserted* into the socket), or it may be pierced and vented (Fig. 5) for the injection technique (the pierced, vented molding shell is placed in the socket first; then impression material is *injected* with

---

Marsha Erickson Guibor, Certified Ocularist, New York, N.Y.

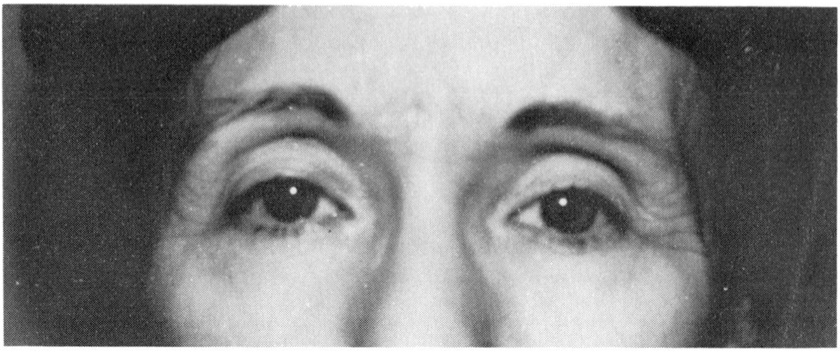

FIG. 1. Patient with bilateral blepharosulcus depression, not a deformity.

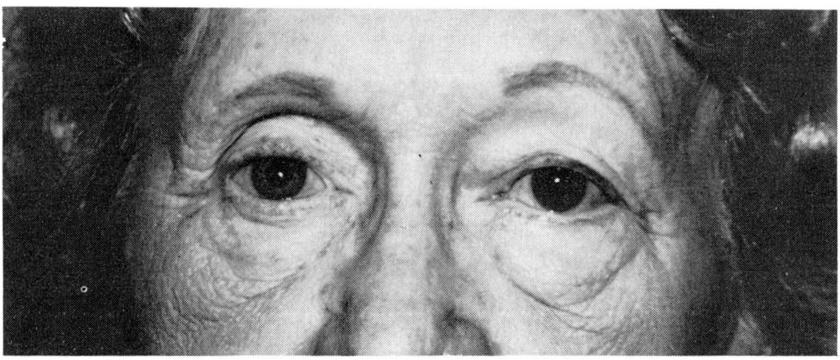

FIG. 2. Patient with unilateral blepharosulcus depression, a deformity.

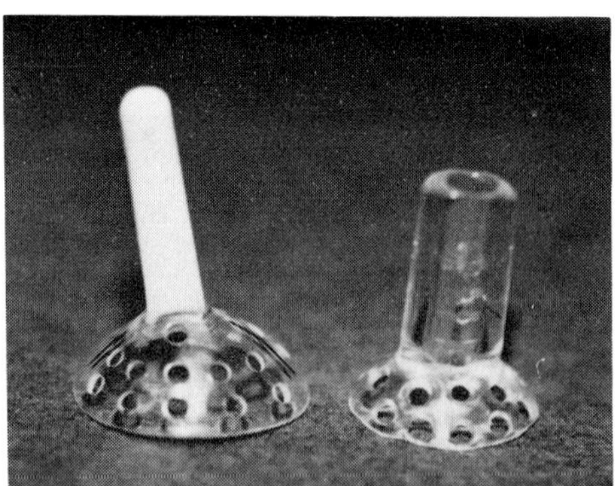

FIG. 3. Conventional impression shells or trays.

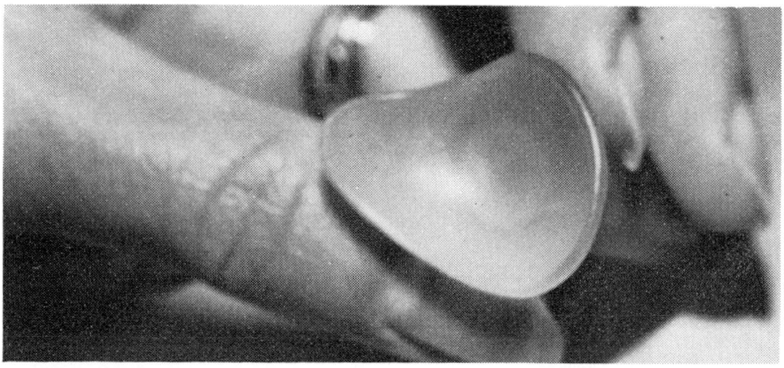

FIG. 4. Custom-made, empirically fitted, wax molding shell for insertion technique.

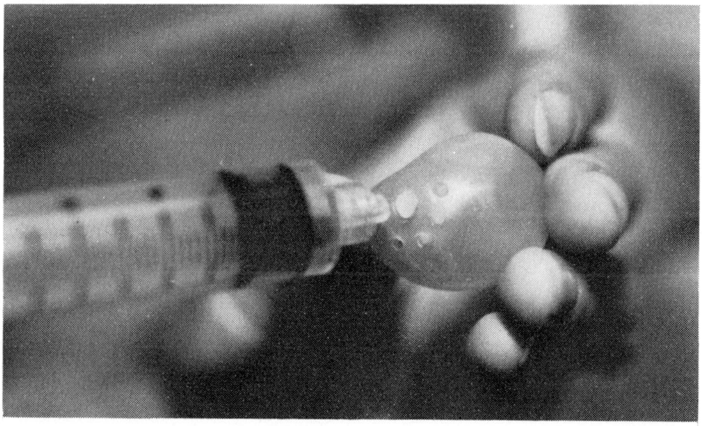

FIG. 5. Custom-made, empirically fitted, wax molding shell for injection technique.

a disposable syringe through the pierced portion of the molding shell, allowing the excess impression material to escape through the vents). The Allen-Webster blepharosulcus-ptosis correction procedure [1] is employed in the custom-made, empirically fitted, wax impression shell (Fig. 6). When it is inserted into the socket without impression material, it very closely approximates the final, desired palpebral fissure and fits securely into the fornices (Fig. 7). This takes advantage of the motility that may originate from the fornices and also prevents gaps that may occur at the medial and lateral canthi on excursion when a conventional impression shell is employed.

In the cross section of an empty socket shown in Figure 8A, one can see that there is a blepharosulcus depression, blepharoptosis and an ectropion of the lower lid; but most important, one can see that the tissue has many folds and that its general shape is nondescript. It is preferable to

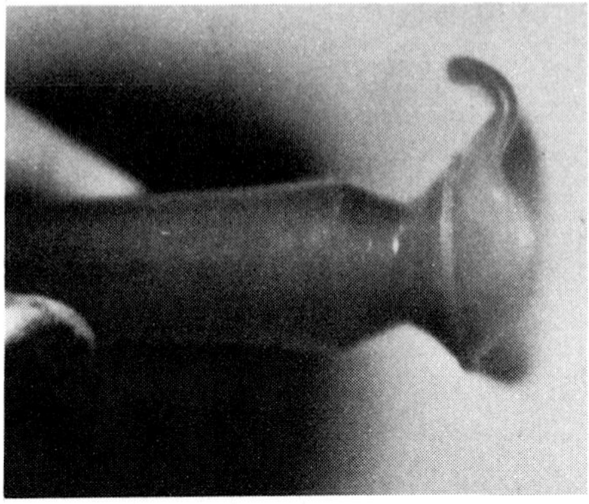

FIG. 6. Blepharosulcus-ptosis correction procedure employed in design of custom-made, wax molding shell.

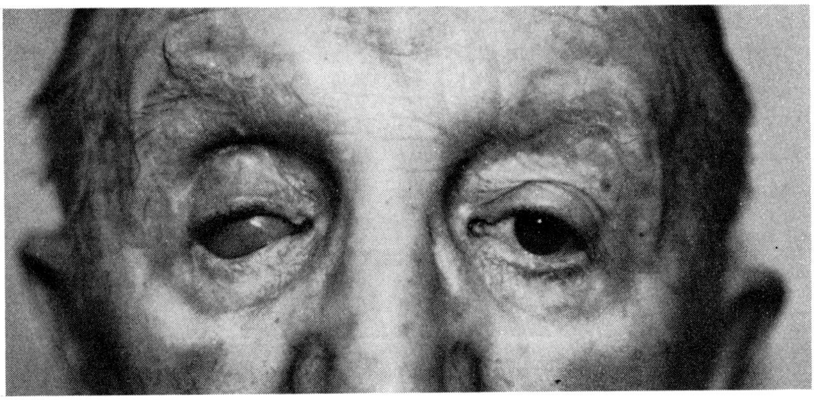

FIG. 7. Wax molding shell, without impression material, approximating desired palpebral fissure.

give this nondescript folded tissue shape and purpose first with an empirically fitted, wax molding shell (Fig. 8B) and then take an impression. With this technique the impression material takes the shape of the tissues and implant *as they exist with the lids in the corrected positions,* while the empirically fitted molding shell assures a secure fit into the fornices. The rounded inferior aspect of the prosthesis (Fig. 9A) places too much of the weight of the prosthesis on the lower lid, forcing it to sag. By changing the shape of the inferior aspect of the prosthesis (Fig. 9B), the weight is removed centrally and redistributed to the areas of the medial and lateral canthi, allowing the lid to be raised. This design should be incorporated into the wax shell.

The impression is taken (Fig. 10), in this instance by the insertion technique, and an accurate impression is yielded (Fig. 11). The impression

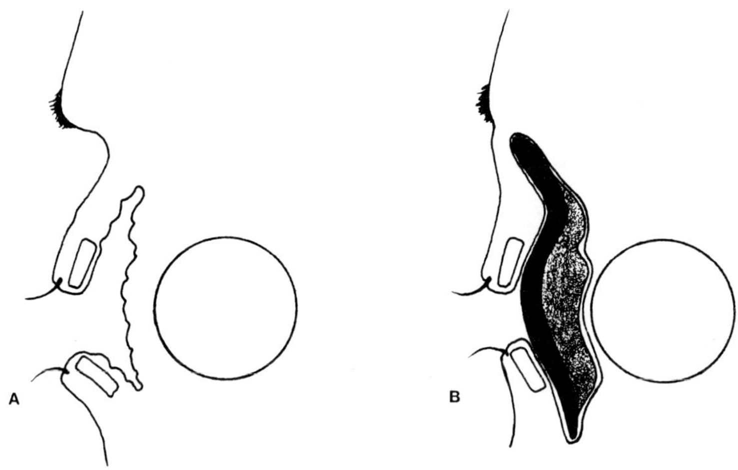

FIG. 8. (A) Cross section of an empty socket depicting blepharosulcus depression, blepharoptosis, lower lid ectropion and tissue folds. (B) Cross section of socket with custom-made, empirically fitted, wax molding shell correcting deformities. Shaded area represents impression material.

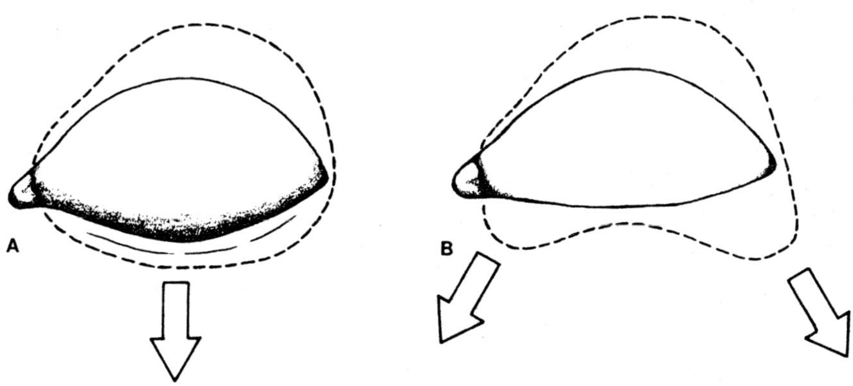

FIG. 9. (A) Inferior aspect of prosthesis too round, causing sagging of lower lid. (B) Shape change of inferior aspect of prosthesis redistributes weight, allowing lid to be raised.

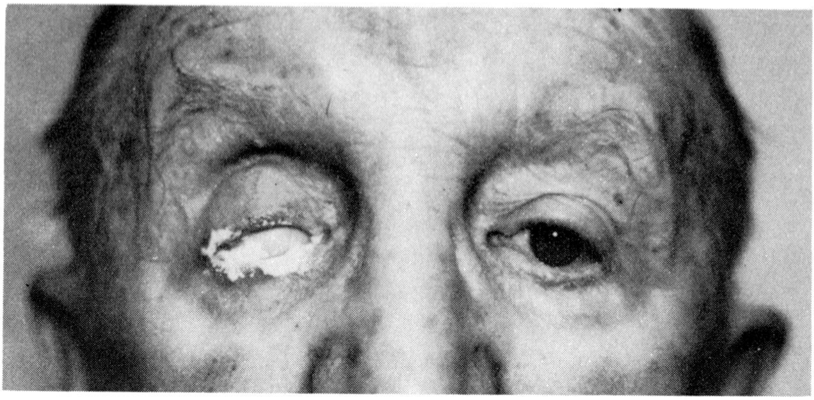

FIG. 10. Impression being taken with custom-made, wax molding shell.

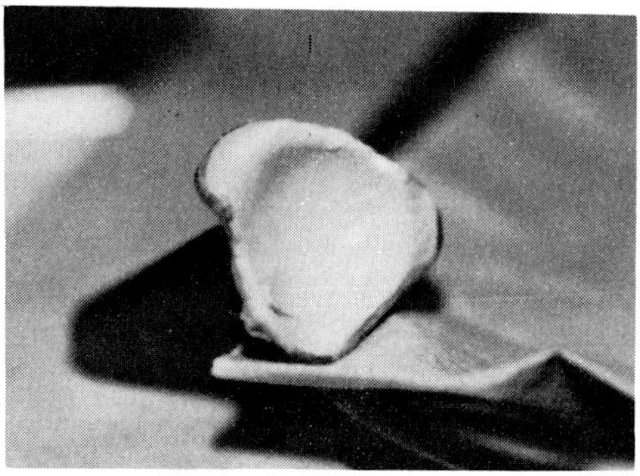

FIG. 11. Actual impression yielded.

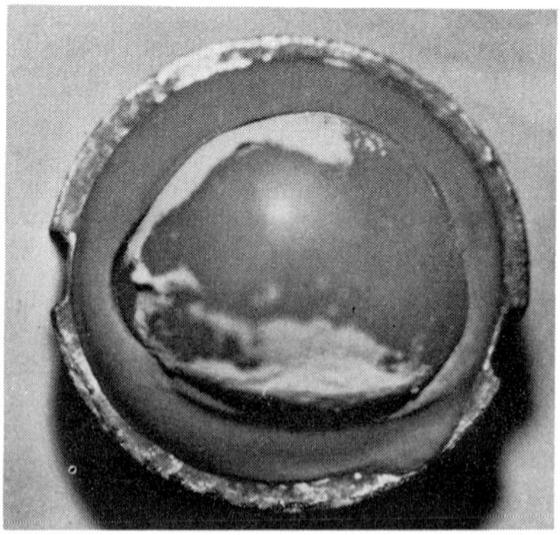

FIG. 12. Impression invested into stone. Note overflow material at superior and inferior aspects of impression.

can then be invested into stone in a flask. If overflow appears on the anterior surface of the final impression (Fig. 12), it should be removed (Fig. 13) as it will only distort the design. The investment into the flask is completed without the encumbrance of a handle or injection receptacle (Compare Fig. 3 with Fig. 14). The bottom half of the cast, which details the posterior portion of the impression, is placed into the cylindrical chamber of the impression duplicator (Fig. 15); white plastic sheet is heated until pliable and placed over the flask. The top of the cylinder is closed tightly and nitrogen gas is forced into the chamber at a pressure of 400 pounds per square inch. In approximately two minutes a duplication of the posterior aspect of the impression will be created (Fig. 16). It may

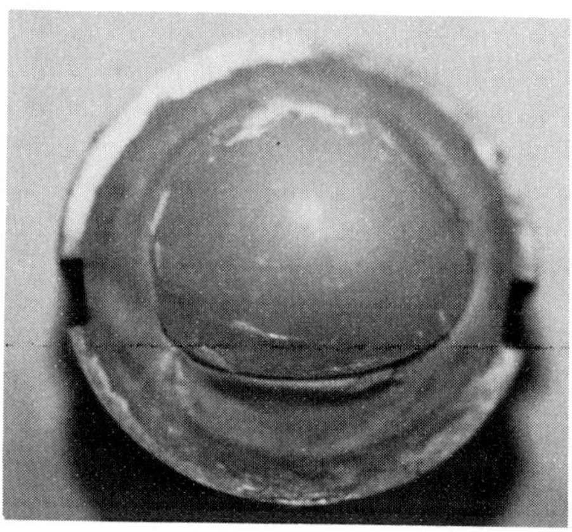

FIG. 13. Overflow impression material removed to prevent distortion of design.

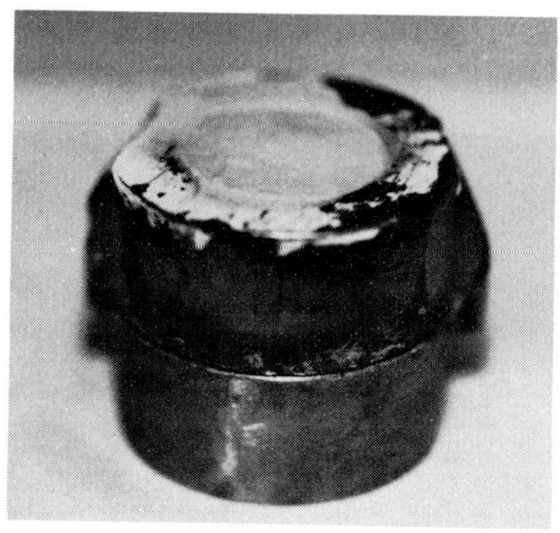

FIG. 14. Completed flask without encumbrance of handle or injection receptacle.

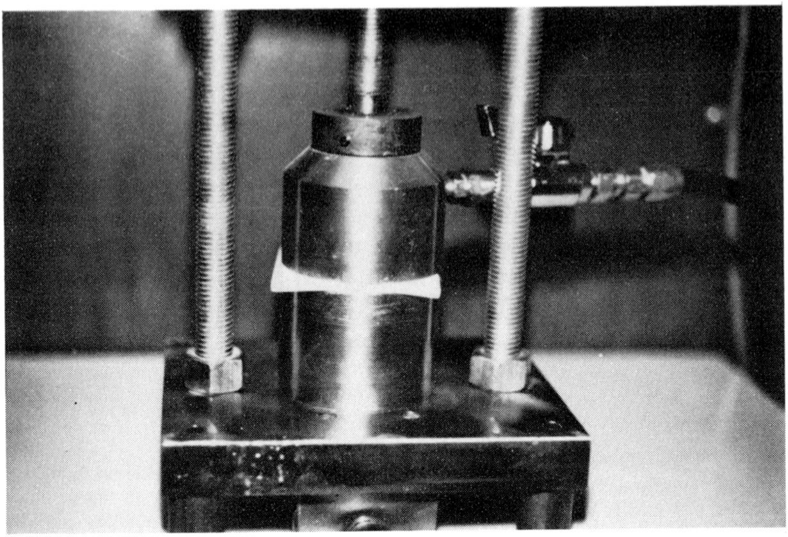

FIG. 15. Impression duplicator.

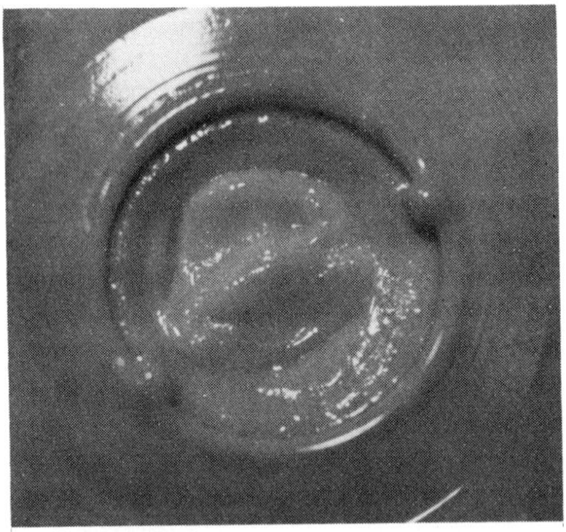

FIG. 16. Plastic duplication of posterior aspect of impression.

be cut out with a bur in the laboratory and used as the base of the prosthesis (Fig. 17). The prosthesis is then completed, duplicating the impression (Fig. 18).

In the photographs of a patient wearing a nonimpression-type conformer (Fig. 19) and the same patient wearing the impression-fitted prosthesis, duplicated by the procedure described above (Fig. 20), one can compare the difference in the blepharosulcus depression, the blepharoptosis and the sagging lower lid.

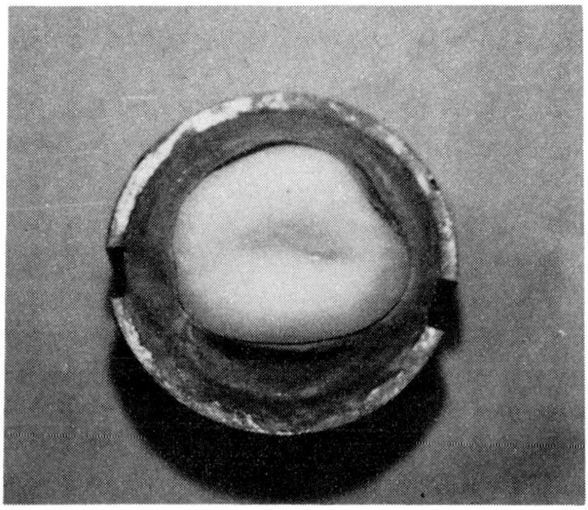

FIG. 17. Plastic duplication cut out for use as back of prosthesis.

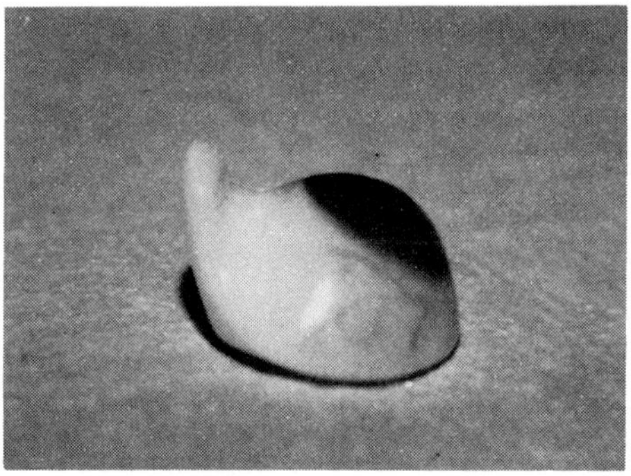

FIG. 18. Prosthesis employing blepharosulcus-ptosis correction principle.

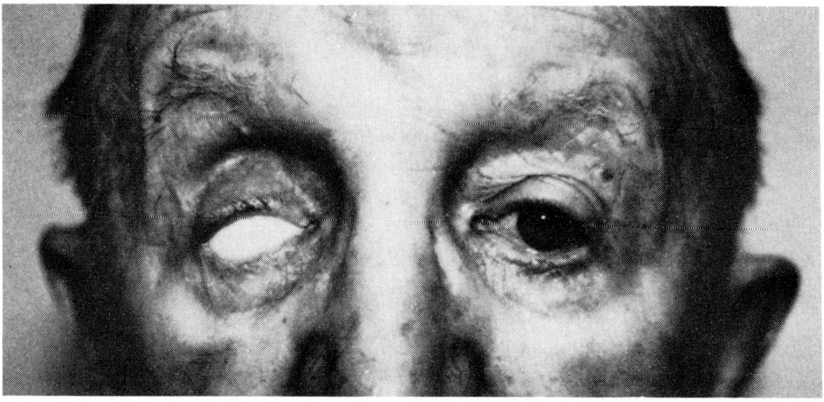

FIG. 19. Patient wearing nonimpression-type conformer.

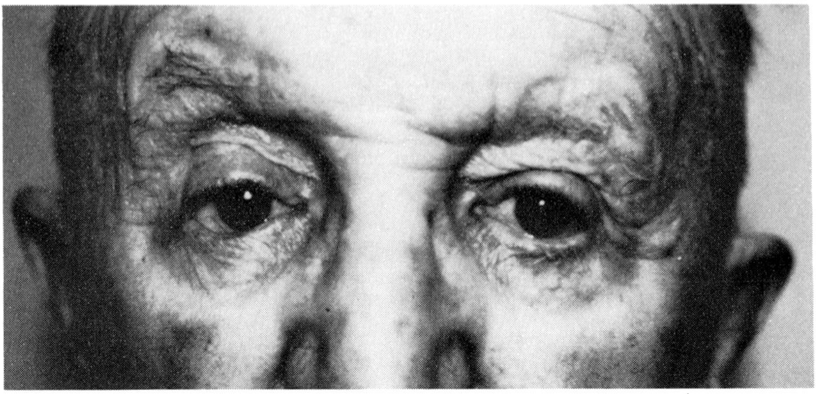

FIG. 20. Patient wearing impression-fitted prosthesis, produced by described procedure.

In summary, a custom-made, empirically fitted, wax shell which corrects anatomic deficiencies of the aging anophthalmic patient, ie, blepharosulcus depression, blepharoptosis and a sagging lower lid, may be used as an impression shell or tray. Used in this manner, it combines the advantages of fitting into the fornices securely and allowing the impression material to take the shape of the tissues and implant as they exist with the lids in the corrected positions, hence offering comfort, cosmesis and maximum motility to the patient.

Acknowledgment

The authoress wishes to extend thanks for inspiration to Dr. Pierre Guibor and Mr. Jack Erickson. Mr. Erickson, a certified ocularist, is equally responsible for the innovation of this technique and duplicating process; without his technical skill it would not have been possible.

Reference

1. Allen, L. and Webster, H.: Modified impression method of artificial eye fitting. Amer. J. Ophthal., 67 (2):189-218, 1969.

Anophthalmic Cosmetic Blepharoplasty

Pierre Guibor, M.D.

Introduction

Blepharoplasty is a term first described by von Graefe [1] in 1818 in reference to lid reconstruction secondary to the resection of palpebral carcinomas. The cosmetic aspects relative to the aging processes were not envisioned by von Graefe. In the 1800s new and creative operations were devised by Goyrand, Morax and others concerning lid reconstruction techniques.

In the early 1900s Elschnig [2], Hotz [3], Fuchs [4], Padgett [5], Spaeth [6] and others started to discuss baggy eyelids, herniated orbital fat, blepharochalasis, lipoma, ptosis, ptosis lipomatosis and a myriad of other terms relative to the current era of cosmetic blepharoplasty.

Rees and Wood-Smith [7] have published an excellent, detailed description of cosmetic blepharoplasty techniques in their recent book, *Cosmetic Facial Surgery*.

The term "cosmetic blepharoplasty" today refers to the resection of skin and/or orbital fat in a symmetrical fashion to reduce the unsightly reflections of age, fatigue and endocrine abnormalities. Cosmetic blepharoplasty has become extremely popular among every class, generation and society of today.

Anophthalmos refers to a person who has had an enucleation or evisceration. This condition may be unilateral or bilateral; however, for discussion purposes, this paper will be limited to the patient with unilateral anophthalmos.

Anophthalmic cosmesis has previously dealt with the correction of enophthalmos, entropion and ectropion, socket reconstruction, ptosis and various other associated abnormalities. The objective here will be to describe the surgical technique of cosmetic blepharoplasty in those patients with anophthalmos who are wearing an artificial eye or cosmetic cover shell.

Pierre Guibor, M.D., Ophthalmologist, New York, N.Y.

The purpose of this surgery should be thoroughly evaluated by the patient, physician and ocularist. The patient desires a more symmetrical facial appearance and especially a more "normal-looking" prosthesis. The enophthalmic appearance of an artificial eye is a main concern to the patient, as are other deformities associated with the loss of an eye. The baggy lids, herniated orbital fat and excessive dermochalasis are usually more pronounced in the normal, seeing-eye side, and the patient usually desires equalization of the lid structures in order to camouflage his anophthalmic condition. The surgeon can accomplish this objective by employing surgical judgment and the techniques available to him (described below). Complications such as retrobulbar hematoma, infection, lagophthalmos, ectropion and chronic blepharitis are more prone to occur in the artificial-eye wearer than in the normal, two-eyed person. The surgeon must employ his ophthalmic knowledge and plastic surgical technique of the highest order, in order to prevent disastrous results in these one-eyed patients who are undergoing elective cosmetic blepharoplasty.

Preoperative Evaluation

Usually the patient who has suffered a permanent loss of an eye, either through cancer, trauma or systemic disease, has already inadvertently experienced the psychological blow of his condition. The previous loss of an eye overshadows the seriousness of a relatively poor result from a cosmetic blepharoplasty. Therefore, the anophthalmic patient tends to be less hypercritical and more accepting of the results of a cosmetic blepharoplasty. However, the patient's expectations, realistic appraisal and psychiatric status are paramount factors to be considered in the anophthalmic patient desiring cosmetic blepharoplasty.

It is essential to rule out specific systemic conditions which masquerade as premature aging of the skin, eyelid edema and herniated orbital fat. The most common disorder is thyroid dysfunction (usually underactive). Hyperthyroidism, renal disease, liver cirrhosis, diabetes, congestive heart failure and ocular allergies are a few important conditions to be considered when examining an anophthalmic blepharoplasty candidate.

The *ophthalmic status* of these patients is extremely important and must be evaluated in detail preoperatively. Impending conditions which may predispose the patient to total blindness should be thoroughly explored. Various vascular diseases, ie, arteriosclerosis, central retinal artery or central retinal vein disease or diabetic retinopathy, may be contraindicating ophthalmic conditions for this type of contemplated surgery. Angle-closure glaucoma may be precipitated by the surgery; therefore, if there is a history compatible with angle-closure glaucoma, the ophthalmologist should perform the required preoperative evaluation. Certainly the surgeon should evaluate the lacrimal production in order to reduce the chances of postoperative dry eye syndrome. Visual acuity, applanation tensions, slit-lamp microscopy and indirect-direct fundoscopy should be performed preoperatively on the normal eye.

The *anophthalmic status* must also be thoroughly evaluated. Again, symmetry should be considered a primary objective and details of preoperative asymmetry should be carefully recorded. Lid positions, hyperophthalmos, hypophthalmos, lateralophthalmos and medial-ophthalmos should be carefully measured and recorded. The condition and design or shape of the patient's prosthesis should be carefully evaluated by the ophthalmologist and the ocularist jointly to determine what influence the prosthesis has upon the herniated orbital fat or baggy lid condition. The design of the prosthesis may be extremely irregular and complex in that the ocularist often attempts to correct superior sulcus depression, enophthalmos and ptosis with creative displacement of tissue by the prosthesis.

Enophthalmos is probably one of the most common abnormalities associated with the anophthalmic state. The surgeon should record the degree of enophthalmos in millimeters with a Hertel exophthalmometer. If the measurements indicate more than 5 mm of anophthalmic enophthalmos, then subperiosteal glass bead implantation or an orbital implant in conjunction with asymmetrical cosmetic blepharoplasty should be employed. However, the majority of patients will respond well to an asymmetrical resection of lid skin and fat in those cases with minimal enophthalmos. When the anophthalmic socket is borderline in size, glass beads should never be inserted subperiosteally without first informing the patient that socket reconstruction may be necessary following the correction of the enophthalmos.

Compromised sockets should be corrected prior to any cosmetic blepharoplasty because of the traumatic effect of this reconstructive procedure on the orbital tissues. Implant position and the condition of the overlaying tissues should also be carefully scrutinized prior to cosmetic blepharoplasty. If a migrated implant places pressure inferiorly, there may well be associated herniated orbital fat of the anophthalmic lower lid. Conversely, if there is a superior migration of the implant, there may be an associated sunken lower lid. If an implant is partially extruded or the conjunctiva-Tenon's capsule is extremely thin, scleral grafting, temporalis fascia transplant or socket revision is indicated prior to cosmetic blepharoplasty. Entropion and ectropion may be corrected at the time of cosmetic blepharoplasty; however, it is my feeling that the patient might benefit from a more controlled procedure done in a two-stage technique.

Photographs are extremely important in planning and performing anophthalmic cosmetic blepharoplasty. Black and white prints and Kodachrome transparencies should be obtained preoperatively from a professional medical photographer whenever available. Standard views should be established and the author has established an EPS (Eye Plastic Series). This consists of both eyes gazing up, down and straight; detailed right and left eyes; and full face, eyes open and closed. When the patient is wearing a prosthesis the photographer knows that the artificial eye is to be removed, lids separated and the patient requested to look straight, up, down, left and right for each respective photograph.

It cannot be overemphasized that the anophthalmic patient should benefit from a detailed examination by his ocularist. The surgical interrelationships with the implant-prosthesis are major stumbling blocks to the unwary oculoplastic surgeon. Advice and consultation between the ophthalmologist and ocularist are invaluable aspects of the anophthalmic cosmetic blepharoplasty.

The anophthalmic socket should be irrigated once or twice a day for one month preoperatively. The author prefers simple shower water for three minutes as a routine socket hygiene.

Preoperative antibiotics should be employed in the form of topical Statrol (Alcon) and Inflamase 1% (SMP) four to six times per day for two weeks. Also, systemic ampicillin 250 mg or tetracycline 250 mg (Bristol) four times per day should be started one week preoperatively and continued one week postoperatively.

Surgical Aspects

General anesthesia is preferred because of the unlikely occurrence of an orbital hematoma associated with multiple injections of local anesthesia. However, variations in anesthesiology departments, surgical techniques, patients' systemic diseases or hospital facilities may preclude the use of general anesthesia and require local infiltration of Xylocaine 2% with epinephrine (Astra).

Black and white prints should be located in the operating room for frequent reference during the procedure. Prior to performing the operation, the patient should be prepped, draped and the standard operating room procedure utilizing pHisoHex (Winthrop) and Betadine Scrub (Purdue Frederick) employed. Socket irrigation should be performed with copious amounts of normal saline followed by Garamycin (Schering) topically into the normal eye and socket. The prosthesis should be left in place throughout the operation.

There are some special considerations when performing a cosmetic blepharoplasty on an anophthalmic patient as previously outlined. The author prefers to perform surgery on the anophthalmic side first in order to evaluate the minimal amounts of lid skin and fat to be resected. Overcorrection on the anophthalmic side can easily be a major complication. Horizontal shortening of the lower lid of the anophthalmic side is almost routine. The amount of upper lid skin resected on the anophthalmic side is usually less than on the opposite, normal side. Subperiosteal glass bead implantation on the anophthalmic side reduces the amount of fat to be removed and skin to be resected from that side and therefore should be done first.

Excess upper lid skin is resected after an ellipse is drawn on the lid with brilliant green ink (Figs. 1-5). The lower incision of the uppper lid skin resection is placed in a curvilinear relationship just above the ciliary margin and below the supratarsal fold. With time this lower incision migrates superiorly and neatly camouflages itself in the supratarsal fold. With a forceps the surgeon grasps the upper lid skin, prior to any local infiltration, and adjusts the level of the upper incision so that the eye is open approximately 3-4 mm. Again, less skin is usually required to be resected from the upper lid of the anophthalmic side (Fig. 2). The medial to lateral skin resection is performed with a Bard-Parker No. 15 blade (Fig. 3). The medial fat pocket is usually reduced on the anophthalmic side and less fat removal is required. Following light pressure on the globe or

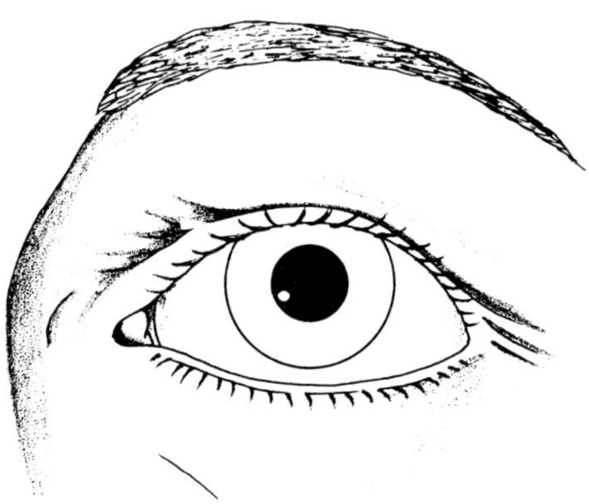

FIG. 1. Excess upper lid skin.

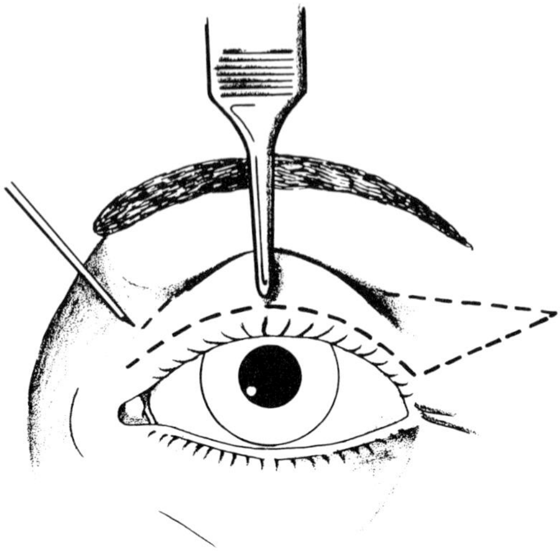

FIG. 2. Marking of upper lid skin resection so that lid is open 3-4 mm.

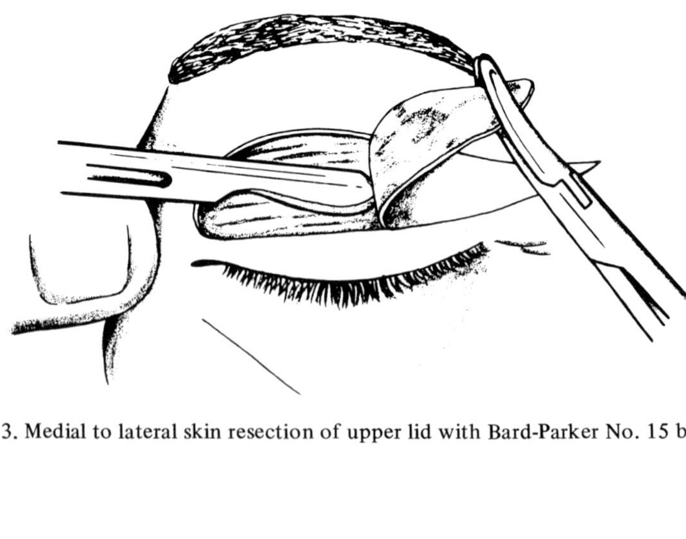

FIG. 3. Medial to lateral skin resection of upper lid with Bard-Parker No. 15 blade.

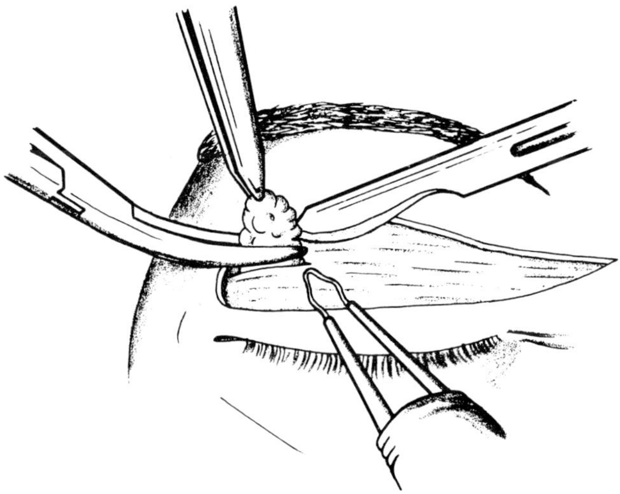

FIG. 4. Excess medial pocket of fat clamped, resected and cauterized.

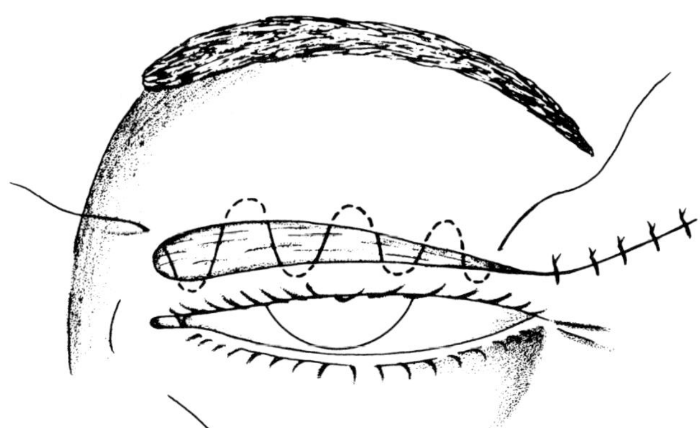

FIG. 5. Continuous subdermal closure with 5-0 nylon and interrupted 6-0 Dexon cutaneous sutures.

prosthesis, this medial pocket of fat is easily visualized and opened with a spring-handled scissors. The appropriate fat is then clamped, incised and cauterized (Fig. 4). The orbital septum is *not* sutured. Skin closure is performed following careful and meticulous applications of cautery to bleeders. A continuous 5-0 nylon suture is first placed subdermally and then 6-0 Dexon approximates the epithelium in an interrupted fashion (Fig. 5). The interrupted sutures are removed on the third or fourth postoperative day, and the subdermal pull-out sutures of 5-0 nylon are removed in five to seven days.

The skin-muscle flap technique is the author's preferred method for removal of lower lid fat pockets which are three in number: central, medial and lateral. On some patients with excess skin this has been an excellent technique; however, when there is increased wrinkling in the lower lid it is desirable to use a skin flap resection primarily. In either case, the infralash incision is made along a parallel line 2 mm below the lower lashes and extends laterally parallel to the lateral canthal tendon. Seventy-five percent of the time a skin-muscle flap is employed in the lower lid cosmetic blepharoplasty (Figs. 6-10). The incision is made from the medial to lateral aspect of the lower lid through the skin and muscle down to the pretarsal tissues (Fig. 6). With rake retractors inserted at the edges, the dissection is carried down off the tarsal plate onto the conjunctival tissue (Fig. 7). As the dissection is carried inferiorly the orbital septum with its underlying pockets of fat becomes evident. With a spring-handled scissors the orbital fat is released and allowed to prolapse

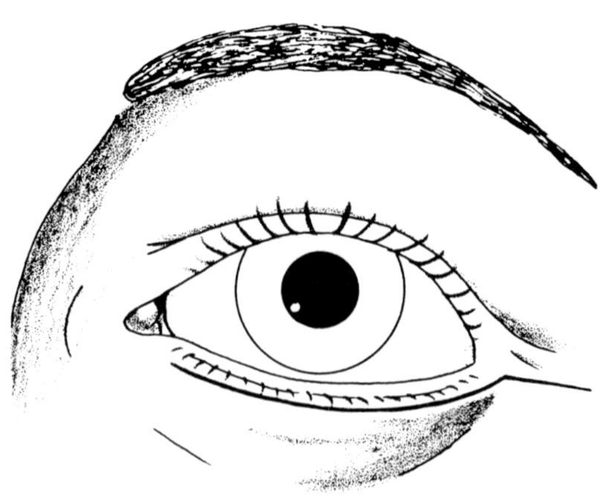

FIG. 6. Infralash razor blade incision to develop skin-muscle flap.

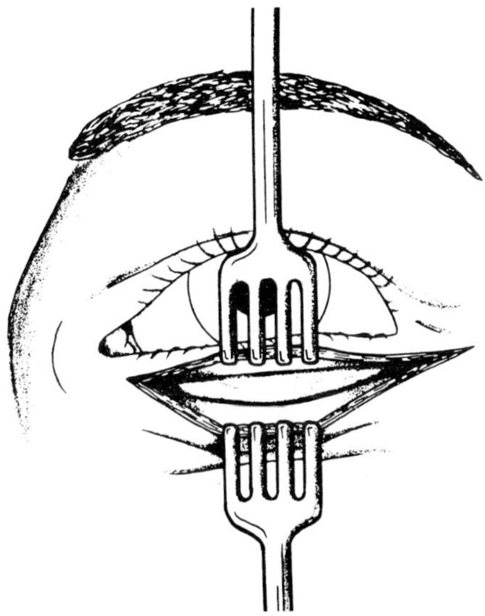

FIG. 7. Inferior dissection of skin-muscle flap to tarsus and conjunctiva.

through the incision, with the surgeon applying gentle pressure on the prosthesis or globe (Fig. 8). It is important that the surgeon never "dive" into the orbital fat and put excessive tension on the fat globules. The orbital fat is then clamped with a hemostat and incised with a Bard-Parker No. 15 blade and cautery is applied (Fig. 9). The surgeon must be sure not to cauterize the skin margins inadvertently. Poor wound healing and scarring result from excessive or inadvertent cautery applications. Recently the thermal-type cautery has replaced the electrocurrent Bove-type cautery in cosmetic blepharoplasty. The orbital septum does not require suturing, and several complications have been seen recently from suture reactions around septal repair areas in cosmetic blepharoplasty. The skin-muscle flap is then draped back to its original location and sutured in place with full-thickness skin-muscle closure of 6-0 Dexon, silk or nylon (Fig. 10). The amount of fat removed on the anophthalmic side is usually less than on the normal side. It is important to compare both lower lids regarding the amount of fat resected, prior to incision closure.

Subperiosteal glass bead implantation reduces the amount of fat resected. However, it is rare to have enophthalmos with a prosthesis and have an associated baggy lower lid; therefore, the most common operations deal with subperiosteal glass bead insertion on the anophthalmic side and a unilateral cosmetic blepharoplasty on the opposite, normal side.

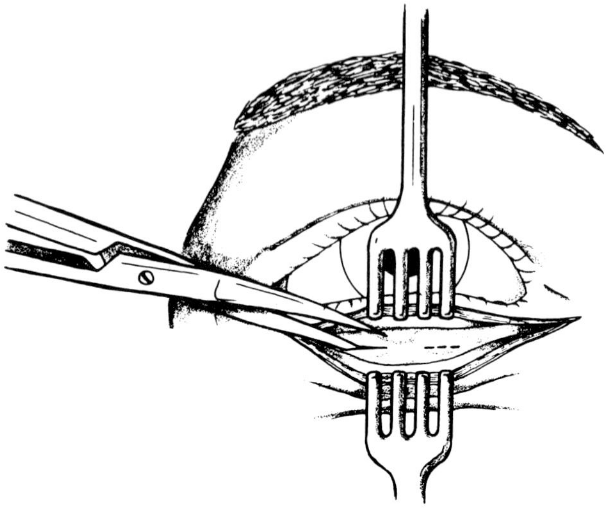

FIG. 8. Dissection through orbital septum into fat pockets.

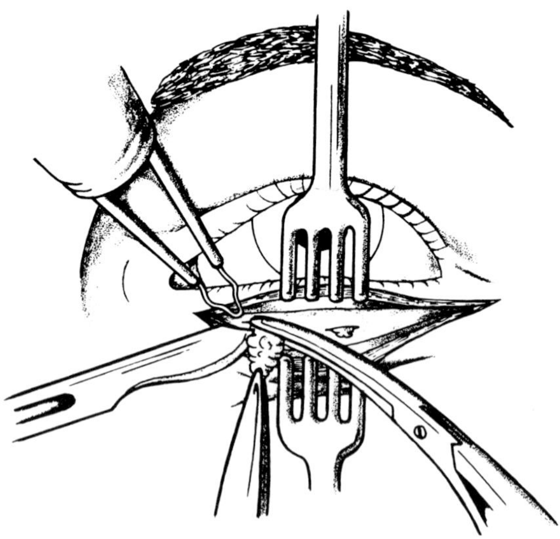

FIG. 9. Herniated orbital fat being clamped, incised and cautery applied *without* orbital septum sutures.

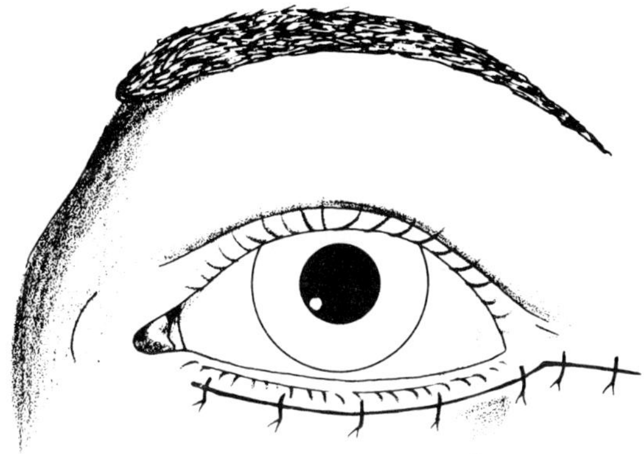

FIG. 10. Lower lid blepharoplasty closure with 6-0 Dexon, silk or nylon.

When doing both upper and lower lids it is essential to close the upper lid incision first, prior to any skin-muscle resection of the lower lid. The reason for this is that when the upper lid incision is closed it actually elevates the lower lid margin, thus automatically shortening the skin-muscle flap.

The skin flap is employed when senile degenerative changes of the lower lid structures are present and wrinkling is an unsightly condition (Fig. 11). The proper amount of tension must be established and excision of skin should be taken laterally instead of just below the lash line. If too much skin is excised from the infralash area of a relaxed lower lid,

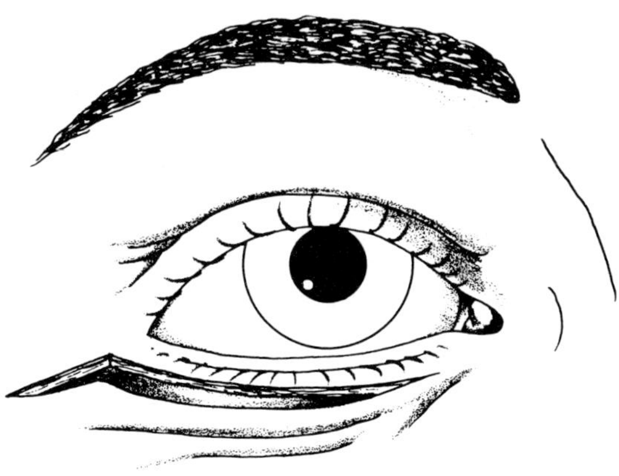

FIG. 11. Relaxed lower lid skin-flap incision.

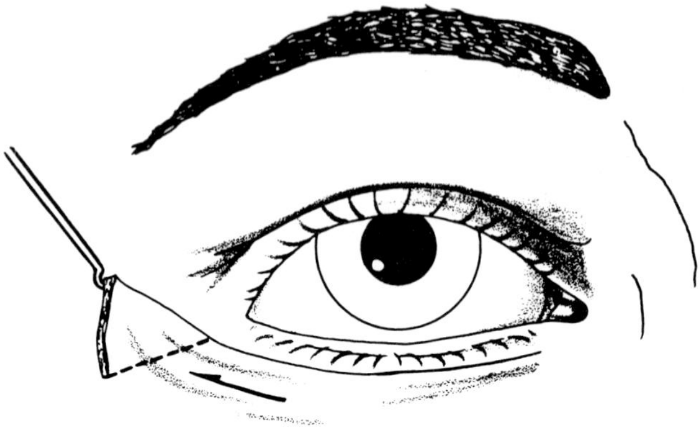

FIG. 12. Proper lateral tension and skin resection from lateral aspect of lower lid blepharoplasty.

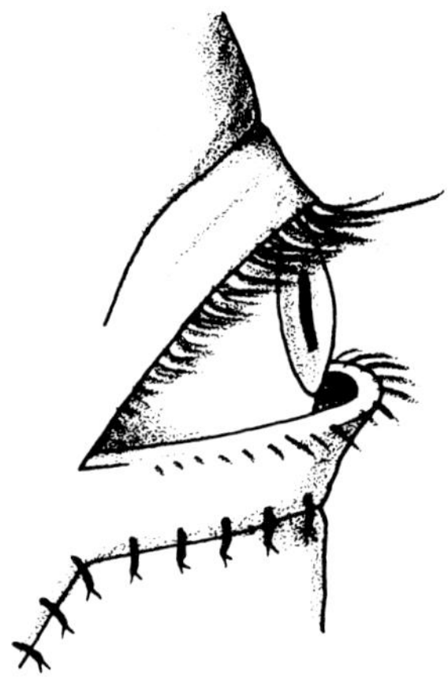

FIG. 13. Excessive lateral tension, excessive skin resection or too inferiorly placed incision of the lower lid blepharoplasty demonstrating secondary ectropion.

ectropion is most certain to occur postoperatively (Fig. 12). The most common complications of cosmetic blepharoplasty are those of post-operative ectropion from excessive skin resection of the lower lid, too low an incision and excessive lateral tension (Fig. 13). The instance of secondary lower lid ectropion is markedly reduced if the surgeon employs a horizontal shortening of the full-thickness lower lid (Fig. 14). The author cannot overemphasize the great importance of the horizontal shortening procedure in the anophthalmic lower lid blepharoplasty. The prosthesis often produces excessive pressure on the lower lid structure and a relaxed lower lid is the rule in association with an artificial eye.

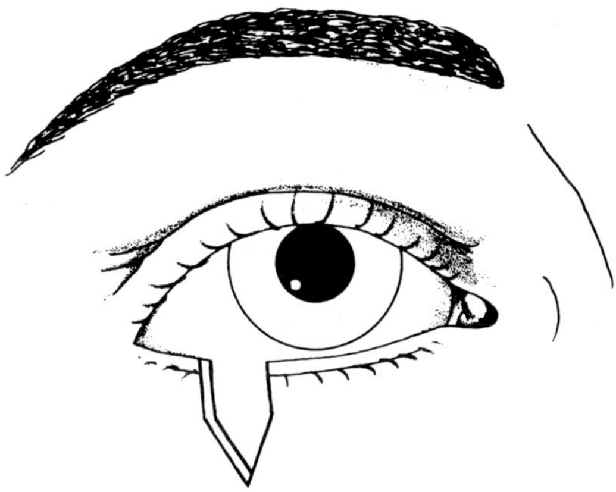

FIG. 14. Horizontal shortening in anophthalmic blepharoplasty.

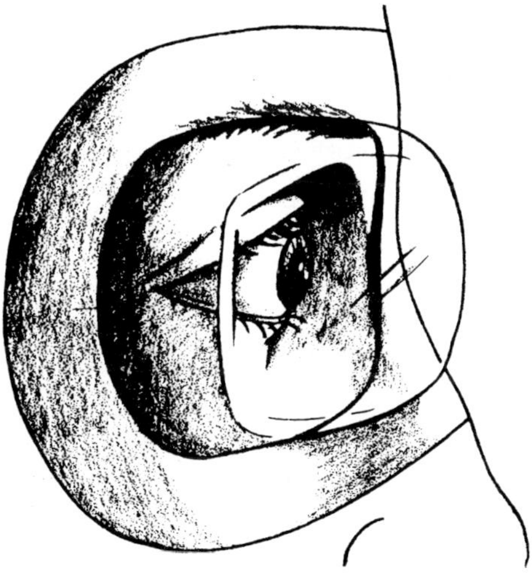

FIG. 15. Expo Bandage-Bubble.

Postoperative Aspects

The exposed normal eye of an anophthalmic patient lends itself to excessive drying, exposure keratopathy and ulceration secondary to the temporary lagophthalmos produced by the upper lid skin resection. The Expo Bandage-Bubble – which is sterile and disposable, provides a moist chamber and prevents drying of the cornea – has been a most rewarding surgical adjunct (Fig. 15).* The bandage remains adherent for 12-24 hours and is then discarded. A sterile Expo Bandage-Bubble is employed at night for sleeping for one month postoperatively. When the patient awakens from the general anesthesia, moist ice compresses are applied directly over the Expo Bandage-Bubble. The interrupted epidermal 6-0 Dexon, silk or nylon sutures are removed in three to four days, and the continuous subdermal 5-0 nylon sutures are removed in five to seven days. It is important to refer the anophthalmic patient to his ocularist immediately postoperatively for evaluation of the prosthesis-socket relationship.

Summary

The anophthalmic patient and surgeon contemplating cosmetic blepharoplasty have many special considerations to be reviewed. Preoperatively it is important to establish the patient's expectations in conjunction with the realistic results contemplated. The psychiatric status, systemic diseases, ophthalmic status and anophthalmic status are vital variables to be analyzed. Prosthetic hygiene, antibiotics and socket irrigation play a major role in reducing the instances of postoperative infection.

The ocularist's role in both preoperative and postoperative care is vitally important. Photographs are essential in planning and performing a cosmetic blepharoplasty on an anophthalmic patient.

Postoperative aspects concerning the Expo Bandage-Bubble, compresses, antibiotics, suture removal and the role of the ocularist cannot be overemphasized.

Acknowledgment

Without the constructive criticisms and technical advice of Mrs. Marsha Guibor and Dr. George P. Guibor this paper would not have met fruition.

References

1. von Graefe, C. F.: De Rhinoplastice. Berlin:Dietrich Reimer, 1818, p. 13.
2. Elschnig, A.: Fetthernien. Sog. "Tranensacke" der Unterlieder. Klin. Mbl. Augenheilk., 84:763, 1930.
3. Hotz, F. C.: Ueber das Wesen und die Operation de Sogenannten Ptosis atonica. Arch. Augenheilk., 9:95, 1880.
4. Fuchs, E.: Ueber Blepharochalasis (Erschlaffung der Lidhaut). Wien. Klin. Wschr., 9:109, 1896.

---

*Manufactured by Procedure Medical Products, Ltd., P. O. Box 229, New York, N. Y 10033; (201) 444-0300.

5. Padgett, E. C. and Stephenson, K. L.: Plastic and Reconstruction Surgery. Springfield:Charles C Thomas, 1948, p. 514.
6. Spaeth, E. B.: The Principles and Practice of Ophthalmic Surgery, 4th ed. Philadelphia:Lea & Febiger, 1948.
7. Rees, T. D. and Wood-Smith, D.: Cosmetic Facial Surgery. Philadelphia:W. B. Saunders Company, 1973.

IV. Free Papers

Blunt Ocular Trauma: Posterior Polar Changes

Howard Schatz, M.D.

The mechanical force of direct, nonpenetrating blunt trauma to the globe sets up concussion waves through the ocular tissues and may result in anatomic disruption in addition to concussion necrosis of these tissues. These changes can affect any one of the layers of the posterior pole, including the retina, pigment epithelium and the choroid. Fluorescein angiography may be extremely helpful in delineating the specific histopathologic effect of the trauma. Thus the prognosis may be determined and therapy appropriately instituted.

Effects on the Retina

Commotio Retinae (Berlin's Edema)

Commotio retinae results from concussion and is thus appropriately termed "concussion edema." The patient notices reduced vision which is proportional to the degree and area of the macula affected. If a large portion of the central macula is markedly involved, vision may be 5/200 or worse. The retina appears cloudy-white with ill-defined margins, usually extending over the entire macula and often to the edges of the posterior pole. When the macula is involved, the fovea appears bright red in contrast to the cloudy-white background. This change occurs fairly rapidly over the first 12 hours after blunt trauma and tends to fade away slowly over the next week or so. By slit-lamp contact lens examination, the inner retina appears thickened with a cherry-red spot in the center of the macula.

The fluorescein angiogram is normal or may even show hypofluorescence as the edema of the retina blocks the choroidal fluorescence, giving a

---

Howard Schatz, M.D., Director, Retina Research Fund, St. Mary's Hospital and Medical Center; Assistant Clinical Professor of Ophthalmology, University of California Medical Center, San Francisco.

dark appearance to the entire posterior pole. Most cases of Berlin's edema eventually resolve with return of good vision. However, a number of patients develop thinning of the retina in the macula which often results in a traumatic macular hole.

Hemorrhage

Hemorrhage occurs as a result of damage to the retinal blood vessels or a true concussion necrosis of the retina. The hemorrhage may locate in several places: superficially, in the vitreous or beneath the internal limiting membrane; in the nerve fiber layer of the retina (flame-shaped hemorrhage); or in the deeper layers of the retina (dot and blot hemorrhage).

Macular Hole

This condition is often the end result of severe trauma in which the inner layers of the retina are most critically affected. The retina loses its cellular structure and becomes edematous and necrotic, and develops into a thin, fibrous band of tissue. The progression of this condition may begin with concussion necrosis (tissue death) or Berlin's edema. The next stages may be cystoid macular edema, leading to a thinning of the anterior wall of the cyst (internal limiting membrane) and, finally, a lamellar hole. In most cases of macular cystoid change and hole, vision is irreversibly reduced.

Hypotony Maculopathy

This lesion appears as a thickening of the retina with horizontal striae (folds) running temporally through the macula from the disk. The condition usually follows a prolonged form of hypotony due to either ciliary body shut-down or a penetrating wound, resulting in rapid loss of intraocular pressure. The vision is usually markedly reduced and a slit-lamp examination demonstrates the thickened, horizontally folded macular retina (Fig. 1).

Fluorescein angiographic findings are usually negative because the retinal vessels in the macula do not leak and there is no abnormal hyper- or hypofluorescence other than leakage of fluorescein from the vessels of the disk in some patients. (Fig. 1).

When the intraocular pressure returns to normal, the folds may disappear. However, in cases in which the globe has been severely damaged and pressure has not normalized, the retinal striae may remain and cause permanently reduced vision. The only therapy is surgical repair in the case of penetrating wounds, in an attempt to restore intraocular pressure.

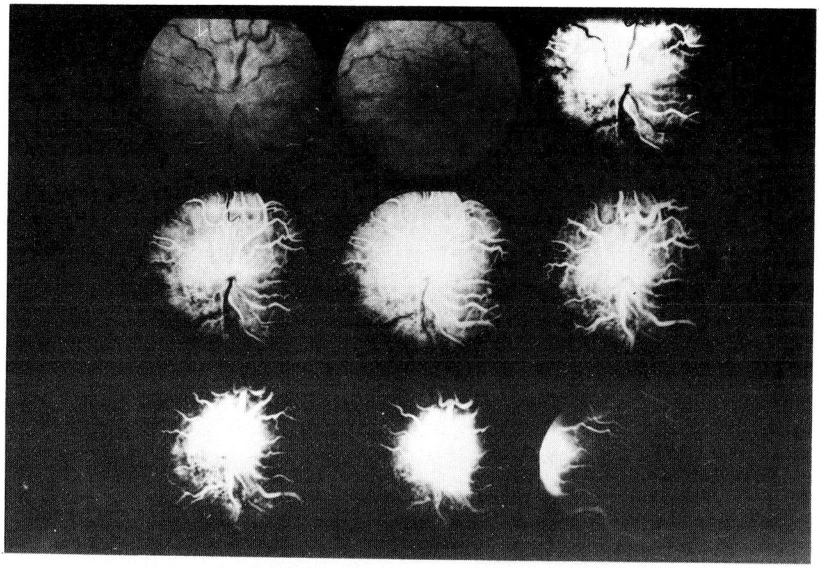

FIG. 1. Hypotony maculopathy. Note the edematous disk and horizontal folds through the macula. The fluorescein angiogram demonstrates marked hyperfluorescence of the disk due to leakage of these vessels. However, there is no leakage from the macular retinal vasculature and the macula remains dark despite the thickened horizontal retinal folds.

Effects on the Pigment Epithelium

Traumatic Pigment Epitheliopathy and Pseudoretinitis Pigmentosa

Traumatic pigment epitheliopathy is a milder form of traumatic pseudoretinitis pigmentosa; each condition may occur after severe, blunt ocular trauma. The appearance of pseudoretinitis pigmentosa is similar to that of hereditary retinitis pigmentosa, although in the traumatic form there may be much more pigment dispersion and migration.

Visual acuity is reduced only if the pigment epithelium in the center of the macula (fovea) is affected. The pigment epithelium surrounding the disc is more often affected, and this gives the appearance of peripapillary atrophy of the pigment epithelium with corresponding pigment epithelial window defect seen on fluorescein angiography. Visual field testing reveals a scotoma, corresponding to the geography of the pigment epithelial atrophy. The peripapillary lesion results in an enlarged blind spot, but since there is no nerve fiber bundle defect visual acuity is not affected.

Occasionally traumatic pigment epitheliopathy is so subtle that even on ophthalmoscopic and slit-lamp examination, the lesion cannot be seen; but on fluorescein angiography it is readily apparent as a pigment epithelial window defect, with easy visualization of the fluorescent choriocapillary flush in the early stages of the angiogram (Fig. 2).

The lesion may take various shapes and forms: it can appear as a ring around the disc or as geographic patches scattered throughout the posterior pole, often affecting the macula in an irregular pattern. Hyperpigmentation may occur, associated with the depigmented geographic lesion (Figs. 2-4).

In addition to the disruption of the pigment epithelium, the photoreceptors are lost (explaining the corresponding field defect); and in more severe cases, choriocapillary atrophy may occur. Further atrophy and pigmentation may develop over a period of time, depending on the degree of trauma. The disease does not affect the inner layers of the retina,

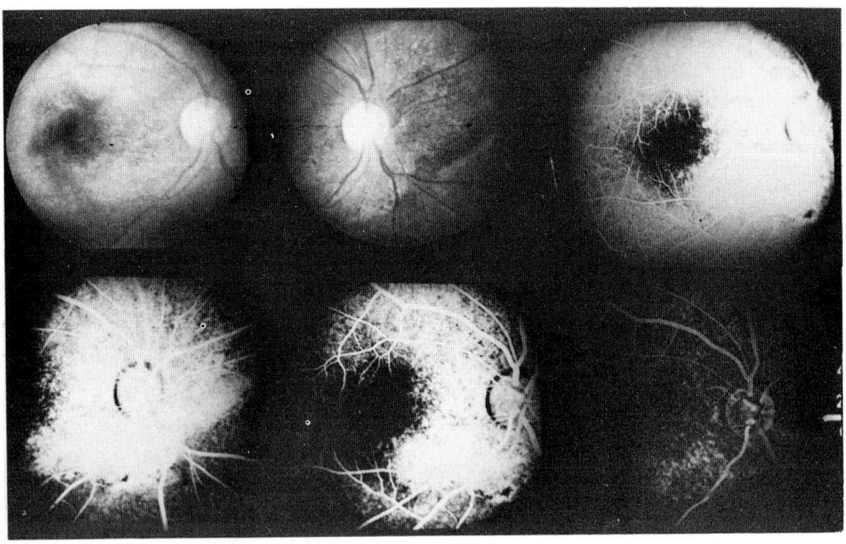

FIG. 2. Traumatic peripapillary pigment epitheliopathy. In the two upper left photos (the ophthalmoscopic view) note the abnormal appearance of the pigment epithelium surrounding the disc and including the papillomacular bundle up to the center of the macula. The remaining photos (the fluorescein angiogram) demonstrate the peripapillary pigment epithelial window defect with early marked hyperfluorescence surrounding the disc and late fading-out of much of this hyperfluorescence – ie, true window defect. There is essentially no hyperpigmentation (pigment migration).

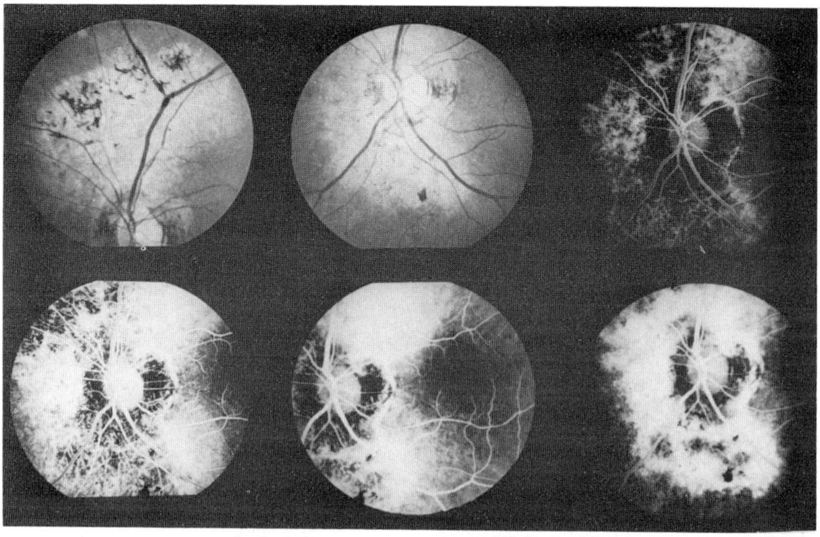

FIG. 3. Traumatic pigment epitheliopathy. Note the depigmentation encircling the left disc. On fluorescein angiography there is marked pigment epithelial window defect in the involved area. In addition, there are a few areas of pigment migration, especially superiorly and around the large retinal vein superiorly. Surrounding the disc there is no window defect because both the pigment epithelium and choriocapillaris are gone.

and thus nerve fiber bundle field defects do not occur. The field defect remains stable despite further pigmentation and atrophic change. There is no known treatment for this condition.

Essentially, traumatic pigment epitheliopathy and pseudoretinitis pigmentosa constitute the extremes of a spectrum of pigment epithelial change secondary to blunt trauma. Such trauma sets off a concussion wave, which possibly shuts down the choriocapillaris, resulting in atrophy of the pigment epithelium; or, there may be a direct concussion necrosis of the pigment epithelium. What follows is marked pigment epithelial disruption and migration, at times culminating in pseudoretinitis pigmentosa in more severe trauma. When there is only a mild change due to less severe trauma, the lesion is most commonly one of pigment epithelial atrophy without any pigment dispersion and migration.

The effects of folds and hemorrhage are discussed in the following section on the choroid.

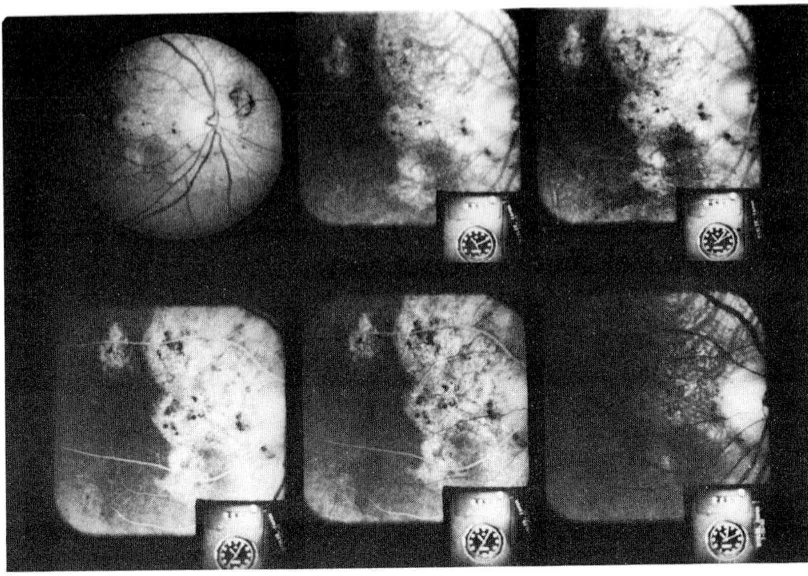

FIG. 4. Traumatic pigment epitheliopathy. Note the total loss of pigment epithelium and choriocapillaris surrounding the disc. On the fluorescein angiogram the large choroidal vessels can be seen in silhouette, and the small amount of remaining choriocapillaris demonstrates marked delay in filling. There is late hyperfluorescent staining of the sclera, easily seen because of the loss of tissue.

Effects on the Choroid

Choroidal Rupture

Blunt trauma may cause one or more posterior polar choroidal ruptures. This lesion is really a rupture of Bruch's membrane with disruption of the continuity of the tissue of the choroid, choriocapillaris and pigment epithelium. The lesion is linear and most frequently concentric to the disc, arching around it, often both nasally and temporally, and occasionally traversing the macula vertically. It is rare to see a linear choroidal rupture which is perpendicular to the disc, but this can occur. Usually hemorrhage initially obscures the appearance of the rupture, and as the hemorrhage clears, the concentric rupture becomes apparent (Figs. 5 and 6). If the choroidal rupture or the resultant hemorrhage involves the macula, vision will be reduced. The nerve fiber layer of the retina is not affected and therefore the visual field abnormalities correspond specifically to the lesion or to the subretinal hemorrhage.

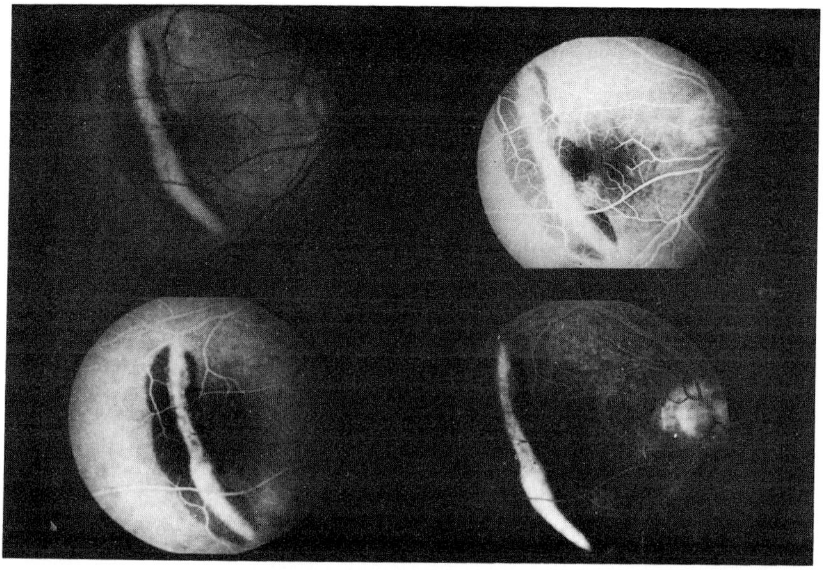

FIG. 5. Choroidal rupture and subretinal hemorrhage. Note the long linear streak concentric to the disc that runs through the temporal edge of the macula. The hemorrhage on each side under the retina is adjacent to the rupture. The rupture demonstrates marked early hyperfluorescence (due to the vascularity) and late staining (due to the scar tissue).

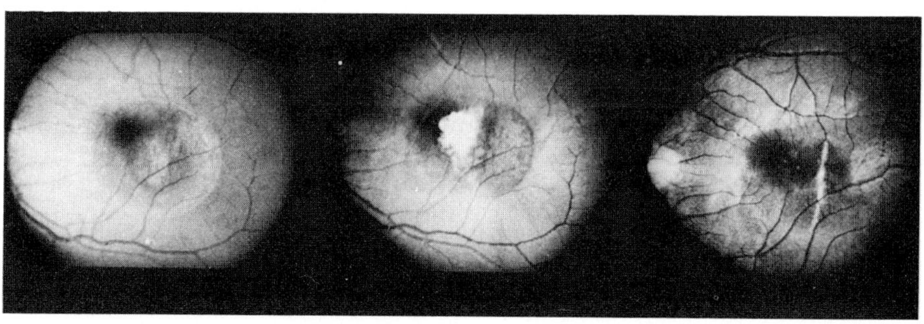

FIG. 6. Subretinal hemorrhage secondary to choroidal rupture. Note the round lesion in the macula in the first photo, taken a few days after blunt trauma. The second photo was taken a few weeks later and demonstrates a yellow lesion made up of the by-products of the resorbing subretinal hemorrhage. The last photo demonstrates a small linear choroidal rupture temporal to the fovea, finally seen because the hemorrhage has resorbed.

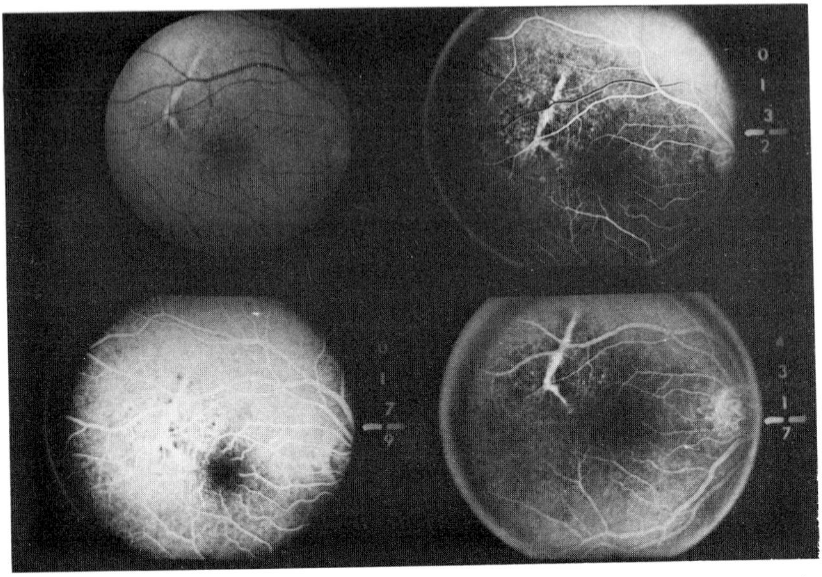

FIG. 7. Old choroidal rupture. Note the linear streak in the superotemporal macula which demonstrates early and later hyperfluorescence. The streak has two short extensions inferiorly. On each side of the rupture are noted pigment epithelial window defects due to the effects of previous hemorrhage and detachment, which have since resorbed.

On fluorescein angiography there is early hyperfluorescence of this lesion, and in the later phases, hyperfluorescent staining of what appears to be a chorioretinal scar (Fig. 7). These lesions resemble angioid streaks, although angioid streaks usually run perpendicular to the disc and emanate from it rather than arching around the disc.

Often there is simply hemorrhage of the choroid, which pushes through the broken Bruch's membrane under the pigment epithelium and, at times, through the pigment epithelium and under the sensory retina. Eventually the hemorrhage clears, leaving a chorioretinal scar in an area of disrupted Bruch's membrane (Fig. 6).

A number of cases have been reported in which the choroidal rupture was associated with, or later developed into, a new subretinal neovascular membrane with sensory retinal detachment, etc. Most often the exacerbated condition of subretinal neovascular membrane formation affects the macula rather than the other areas of the posterior pole and can cause marked visual reduction in a good, seeing eye (Fig. 8).

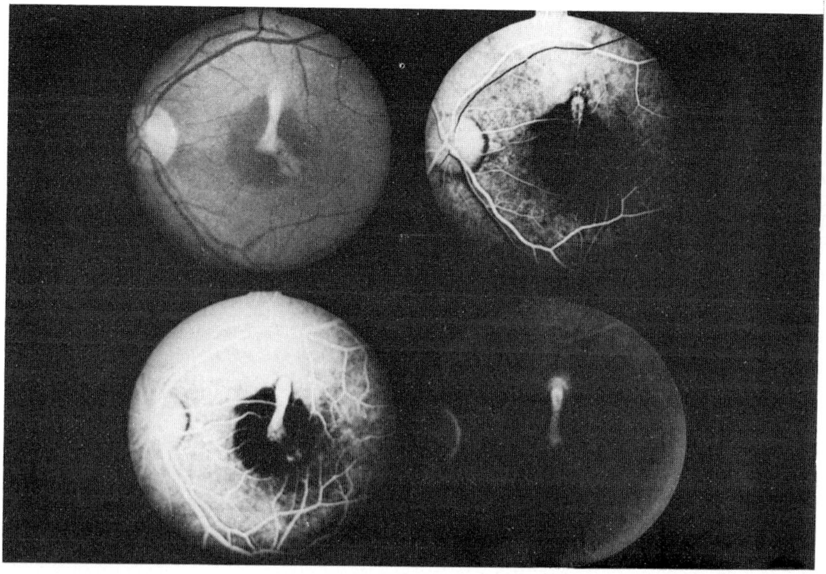

FIG. 8. Choroidal rupture with new subretinal neovascularization and hemorrhage. Note the linear choroidal rupture through the left macula associated with the subretinal hemorrhage. This patient had a traumatic choroidal rupture and later suffered a second blunt trauma to this left eye, resulting in a second episode of hemorrhage and fresh subretinal neovascular membrane formation extending inferotemporally from the previous rupture.

It is the opinion of this author that fresh subretinal neovascular membrane formation emanating from an old choroidal rupture is due to repeated blunt trauma – perhaps *even* less forceful than is usually necessary to effect the initial change (Fig. 8). Patients with choroidal ruptures should take precautions to avoid further blunt trauma, and probably should not rub their eyes or have vigorous scleral depression on ophthalmic examination.

Subretinal neovascularization may be obliterated with argon laser photocoagulation; the sensory retinal detachment can be sealed down and the hemorrhage cleared as a result of obliteration of this membrane.

Choroidal Folds

These have many causes, but in the case of trauma, they usually follow hypotony. Hyper- and hypofluorescence, corresponding to the hills and valleys, respectively, of the folds, distinguish the condition on fluorescein

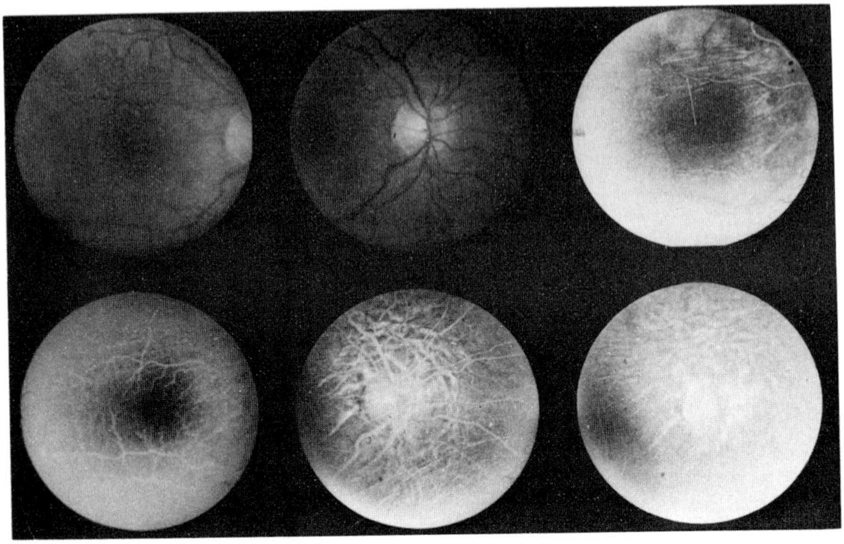

FIG. 9. Old resolved choroidal folds in the eye of a patient who suffered a tennis ball injury with prolonged hypotony one year previously. The intraocular pressure had returned to normal. Note that the black and white photo of the macula and disc appears fairly normal. However, the fluorescein angiogram shows linear folds through the macula and concentric folds around the nasal edge of the disc, with hyperfluorescent "hills" and hypofluorescent "valleys" corresponding to the previous traumatic choroidal folds.

angiography (Fig. 9). In the case of long-standing choroidal folds, the pigment epithelium will have been changed enough so that the linear hyper- and hypofluorescent lines remain even after pressure returns to normal and the folds disappear. Surgical repair may restore intraocular pressure and cause resolution of the folds.

Hemorrhage

Blunt trauma can cause disruption of the choriocapillaris and/or choroidal vessels, resulting in hemorrhage in any layer of the tissues of the fundus. The hemorrhage may remain confined to the choroid or suprachoroidal space (choroidal hemorrhage). Or, the hemorrhage may break through Bruch's membrane and locate under either the pigment epithelium or sensory retina when associated with choroidal rupture (Fig. 10). The hemorrhage may break through the retina and out into the vitreous, also.

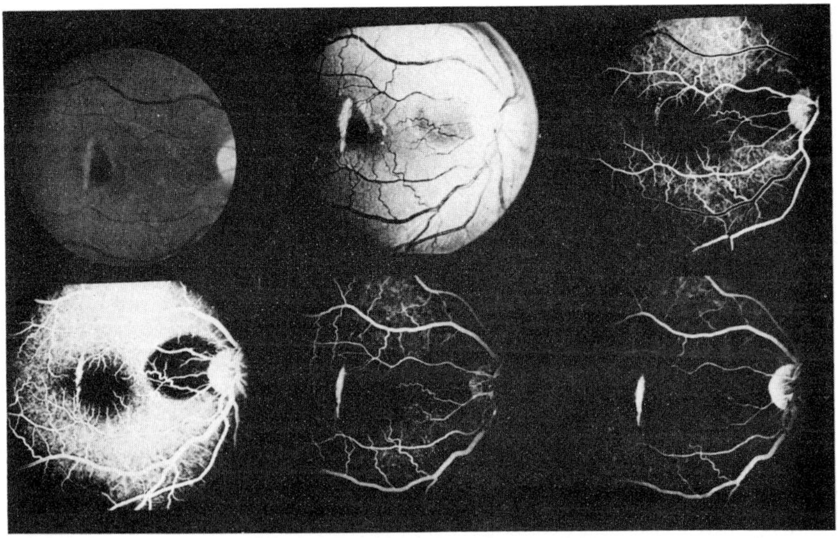

FIG. 10. Peripapillary subpigment epithelial hemorrhage and macular choroidal rupture. Note the choroidal rupture which runs vertically through the temporal edge of the macula with associated subretinal hemorrhage. Adjacent to the disc in the papillomacular bundle is a 1½-disc-diameter, well-demarcated subpigment epithelial hemorrhage. The hemorrhage remains hypofluorescent throughout the angiogram, and the choroidal rupture demonstrates early, lacy (vascular) hyperfluorescence with late staining (due to fibrous tissue).

Acknowledgments

Some of the cases came from the Wilmer Institute, Johns Hopkins Medical School and Dr. A. Edward Maumenee. Thanks are also due to Drs. Tom Burton, Joe Decker, Maurice Robb, David Sachs, Theodore Steinberg and Larry Yannuzzi for referring or contributing cases. The author expresses appreciation to Susan Rabin Schatz and Nancy Esposito for editing, to Claire Ohiyon for photography and to Lorraine Fisher for transcription.

Anophthalmia in South Vietnam

Albert Hornblass, B.A., B.R.E., M.D., F.A.C.S.

Anophthalmia from the Vietnam war represents a serious problem to the medical establishment in the United States but even more so to the civilian population in South Vietnam. During World War II, 1,700 Americans had bilateral enucleations. In the Korean conflict there were 130 totally blind Americans [1]. The Library of Congress has estimated that the ultimate cost of such eye injuries in the Vietnam conflict may reach $4 billion.

The incidence of ocular casualties during wartime has been on the increase. In the American Civil War (1861-1865) eye injuries accounted for 0.5% of all casualties. During the Franco-Prussian War (1870-1871) 0.86% of casualties were eye injuries. In World War II, eye injuries were 2.2% of the total casualties and in the Korean War they were 4.1%. During the Vietnam War [2] ocular injuries accounted for 6.0%-9.0% of the total (Table 1). The eye is only 1/375 of the surface area of the body and only

Table 1. Incidence of Facial and Ocular War Injuries

World War II	2.2%
Korean War	4.1%
Vietnam War	6.0%-9.0%

0.10% of the erect frontal silhouette. The likelihood of severe ocular injury is enhanced by various postures assumed in warfare. For example, although only 25% of the projected body surface is exposed in the prone position, 75% of this area is vulnerable to injury, and the eye comprises a considerable portion of the prone silhouette. The high-velocity fragment missiles used during the Vietnam War accounted for most of the serious eye injuries and a high number of anophthalmic patients [3].

A total of 163 eye injuries were treated by the author in the II Corps of South Vietnam during 1969-1970. Ninety-four had ocular injuries only

Albert Hornblass, B.A., B.R.E., M.D., F.A.C.S., Division of Ophthalmology, Department of Surgery, State University of New York, Downstate Medical Center, Brooklyn, and The Manhattan Eye, Ear and Throat Hospital, New York City.

Table 2. Ocular War Injuries – Pleiku, South Vietnam (1969-1970)

Total	163 Eye injuries
	94 Eye only
	69 Eye and ocular adnexa

Table 3. Nationality of Patients with Eye Injuries

United States	62
Montangard	53
South Vietnamese	47
Cambodian	1

Table 4. Incidence of Ruptured Globes

United States	24
Montangard	34
Vietnamese	35
Cambodian	2
Total	95

Table 5. Incidence of Repair of Ruptured Globes

	Number	*Percent*
Repaired	58	61
Enucleated	32	34
Eviscerated	5	5
Total	95	

Table 6. Percentage of Repair by Nationality

United States	66%
Vietnamese	63%
Montangard	53%
Cambodian	100% (only 2 cases)

and 69 had eye and ocular adnexal injuries (Table 2). Of these patients 62 were U.S. citizens, 53 were Montangards or the local mountain people, 47 were South Vietnamese and 1 was Cambodian (Table 3). There was a total of 95 ruptured globes: 24 were U.S. soldiers, 34 were Montangards, 35 Vietnamese and 2 Cambodians (Table 4). Of these, 58 (61%) were repaired, 32 (34%) were enucleated and 5 (5%) were eviscerated (Table 5).

An attempt was made to repair all eyes. Sixty-six percent of the American, 63% of the South Vietnamese and 53% of the Montangards had successful repair of their ruptured globes (Table 6). The slightly better American percentage may be due to quicker evacuation and better general health. However, it should be noted that the percentage of successful ocular repair has only slightly improved since World War II [4] and the Korean War [5] when approximately one third of ruptured globes resulted in an enucleation. The difference in this war was that more people with severe injuries have been saved due to rapid helicopter evacuation [6] and greater life-saving measures (Figs. 1 and 2).

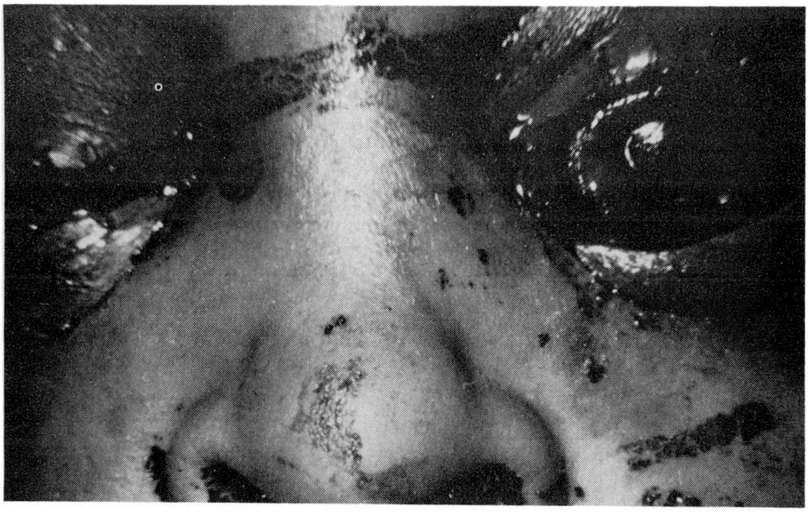

FIG. 1. An American sergeant with a sucking chest wound who survived to the hospital. The left eye shows marked proptosis and subconjunctival hemorrhage, and there is a Le Fort I-bilateral malar fracture.

Fragment-type missiles accounted for 80% of eye wounds. The most common source was a blast injury, ie, rocket (Figs. 3 and 4), mortar and mine (Table 7, Figs. 5-7).

In the Franco-Prussian War 56% of eye injuries resulted in sympathetic ophthalmia; the incidence in the Vietnam War, to my knowledge, is 0. This statistic adds support to the doctine of repairing every eye that is repairable regardless of the visual status of the eye [7, 8].

Associated injuries with ruptured globes were common [9] – 15% of patients had intracranial fragments (Fig. 8) and 20% had fractures of the orbit.

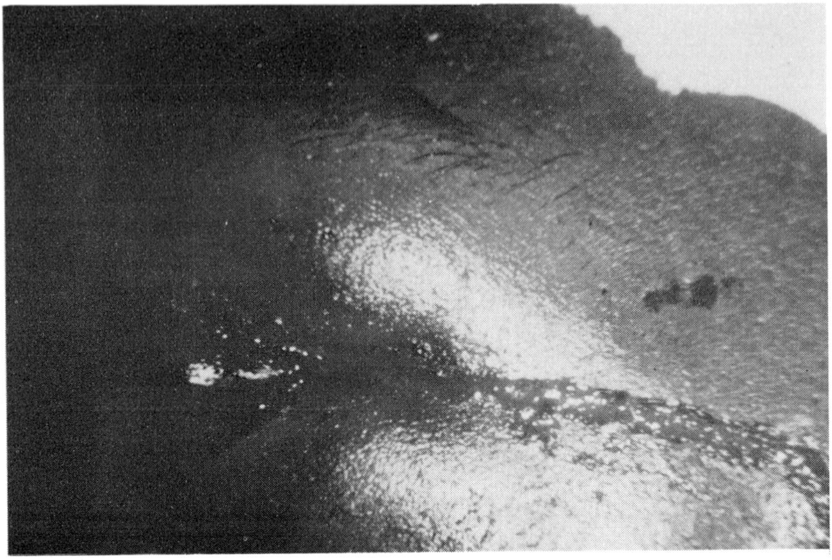

FIG. 2. Lateral view of soldier injured by blast injury. Patient survived severe chest injury. Vitreous hemorrhage began to show some dissolution after several months.

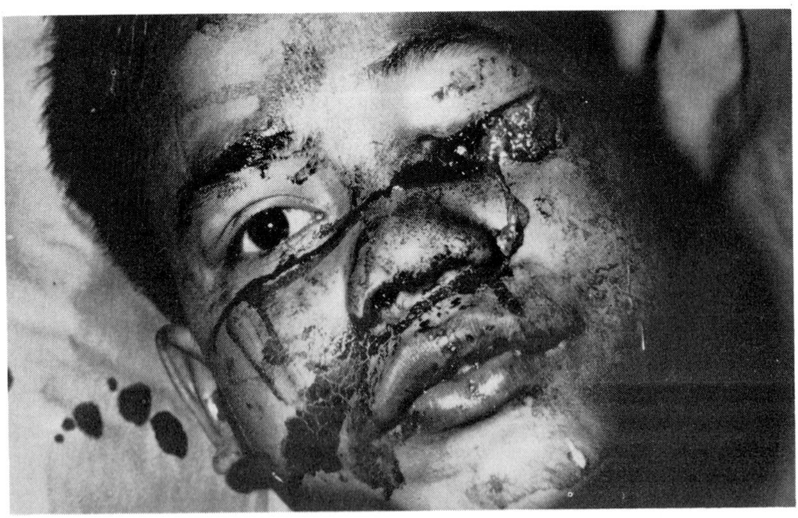

FIG. 3. Rocket injury to a 19-year-old Montangard soldier shows avulsion of left lower lid.

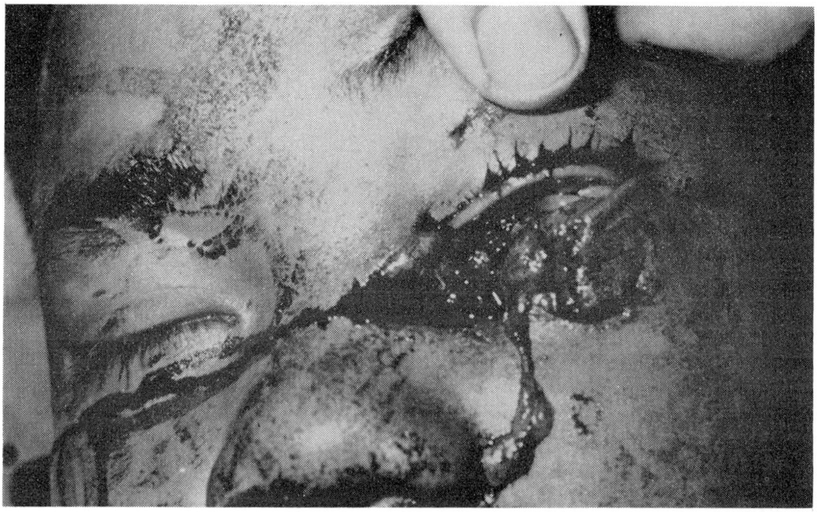

FIG. 4. Closer view of left orbit of the 19-year-old Montangard soldier reveals a complete rupture of the left globe. Enucleation with insertion of a 16-mm glass implant was performed.

Table 7. Sources of Ocular Injuries, 1969-1970

Cause	*Number*
Rocket	39
Mortar	37
Mine	19
Unknown cause	18
Bullet	9
Grenade	7
Pungie sticks	7
Bomb	6
Helicopter crashes	5
Knife	3
Trip flares	3
Rope, wire, satchel charge	1
Sulfuric acid	1
Booby traps	1

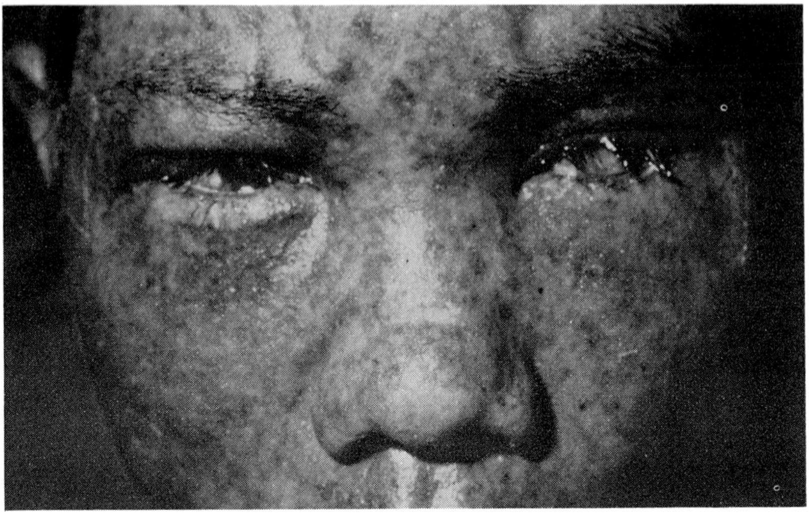

FIG. 5. South Vietnamese, 23-year-old soldier had a mine explode, rupturing left globe and requiring enucleation. Right eye and rest of face are peppered with foreign bodies.

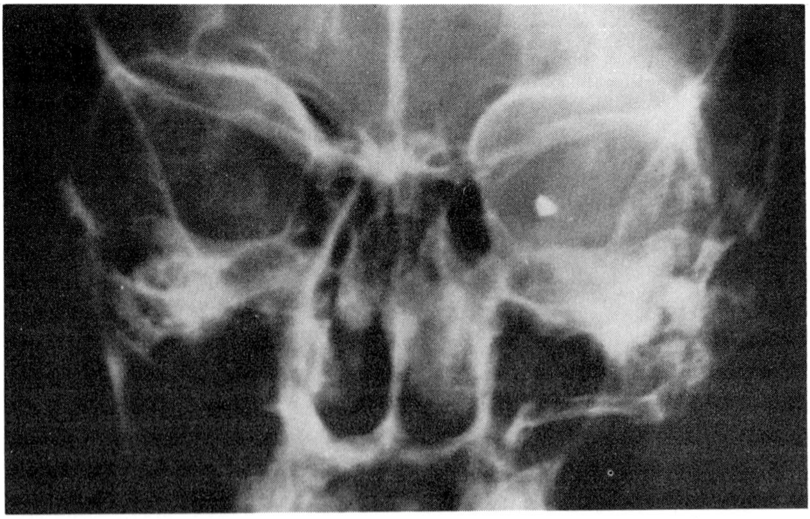

FIG. 6. Fragment from rocket pierced left eye of a 24-year-old American sergeant (AP view).

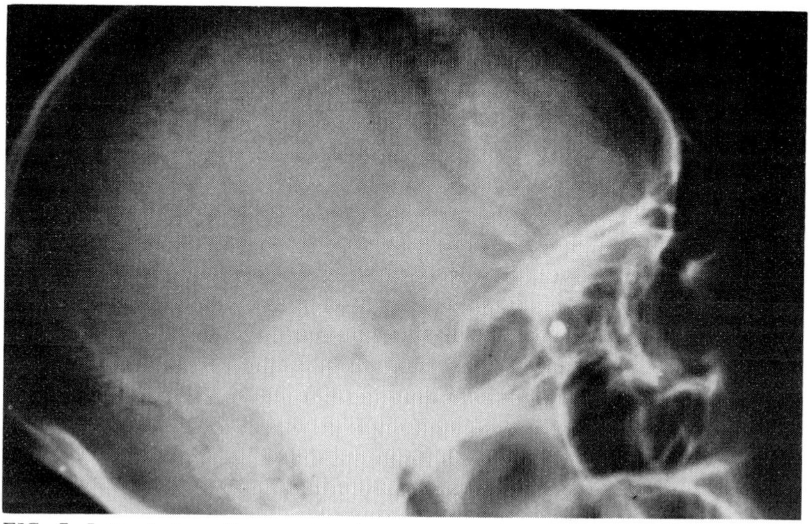

FIG. 7. Lateral view. Fragment is situated at apex of orbit but did not enter the cranium.

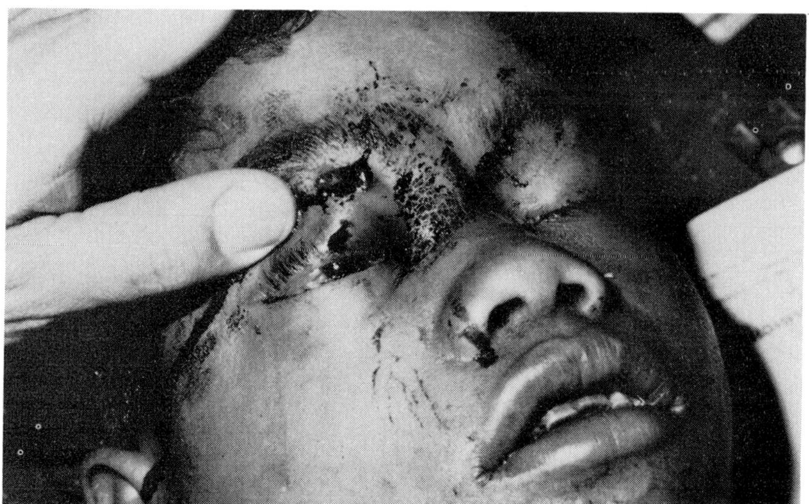

FIG. 8. Mortar injury to Montangard soldier caused severe posterior laceration of right globe. Fragment entered skull, requiring a craniotomy.

Early evacuation with a helicopter, immediate treatment with systemic antibiotics and surgery by a trained ophthalmologist were necessary for successful treatment (Fig. 9). A glass or silicone ball implant averaging 16 to 18 mm was inserted in every case where the removal of the eye was indicated. Overlapping of extraocular muscles was attempted, but frequently this was impossible, particularly when a large fragment destroyed most of the orbital contents (Fig. 10). Every attempt was made to preserve all ocular tissue, particularly the conjunctiva. The largest conformer possible was used to retain the fornices without creating tension on wound closure lines. All eye surgery was performed at an evacuation hospital at the front. There was one case of an implant extruding in an eviscerated eye (Fig. 11). The implant was too large and caused pressure necrosis of the cornea.

To prevent implant extrusion one depends upon:

1. Early surgical intervention.
2. Satisfactory wound toilet.
3. Hemostasis (hot saline packs, pressure patches).
4. Preservation of all extraocular tissue.
5. Adequate implant volume without creating tension in the overlaying Tenon's capsule.
6. At least a two-layer closure.

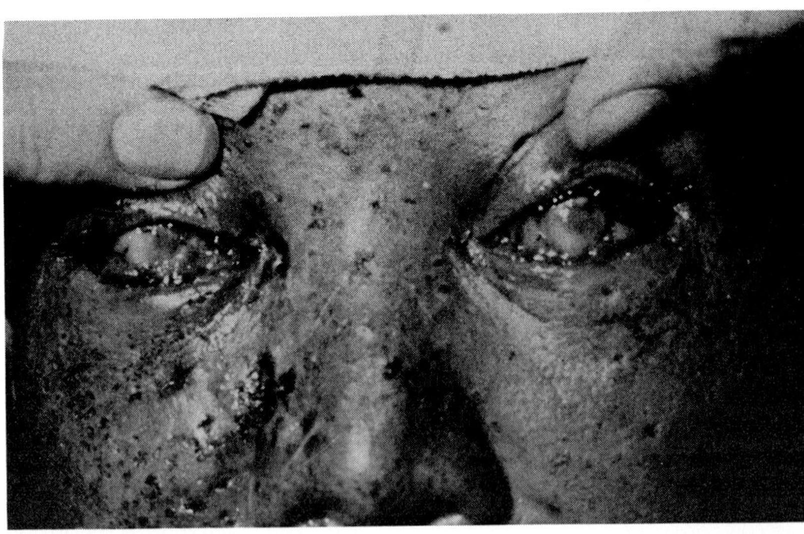

FIG. 9. A South Vietnamese woman was hit with rocket fragments. She was not treated until four days after the attack. Note bilateral panophthalmitis. Right eye injury resulted in evisceration.

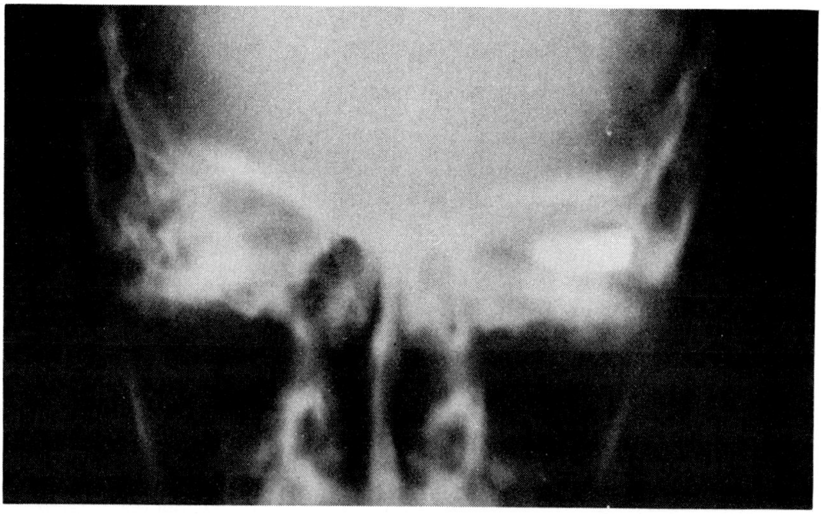

FIG. 10. AP view. Large-size mortar fragments resulted in complete destruction of the globe.

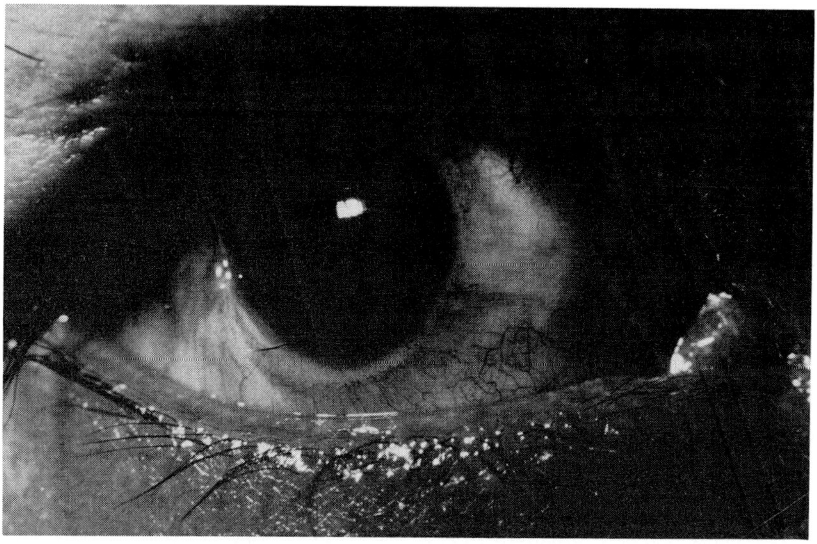

FIG. 11. Glass implant is clearly seen as cornea completely necrosed from pressure in a 20-year-old South Vietnamese soldier.

7. Adequate tissue overlap and secure closure over the implant. (I prefer a Mersiline suture for Tenon's capsule in a purse-string technique.)
8. Horizontal conjunctival closure with preservation of conjunctiva.
9. Systemic and local antibiotics.
10. Irrigation of orbit with sub-Tenon's antibiotics.

The management of war injuries involves a team approach which should include an ophthalmic surgeon, neurosurgeon, maxillofacial surgeon and a plastic surgeon. The care of the anophthalmic veteran involves a team effort as well. It should include the ophthalmologist, ocularist, occupational therapist, psychologist and social worker.

The problem of anophthalmia in South Vietnam remains a serious one. A person who is blind in addition to his handicap is socially ostracized. In various villages he is no longer called by his name but is called "Blind Man." I operated on several young girls with shrunken sockets and fitted them with prostheses. Before they were able to wear an ocular prosthesis no one would marry them. One young girl was married only two months after the insertion of her prosthesis (Figs. 12 and 13). I did not meet a single ocularist in II Corps of South Vietnam and was forced to rely on my friends for old discarded prostheses to fit the native population (Fig. 14). Thousands of Vietnamese are blind today. Most of them do not have ocular prostheses and will be social pariahs.

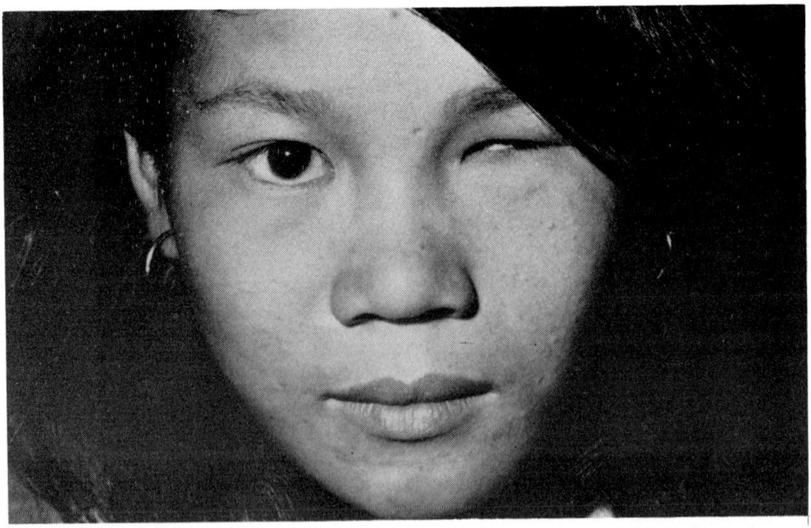

FIG. 12. A 19-year-old South Vietnamese girl with a shrunken postenucleated socket.

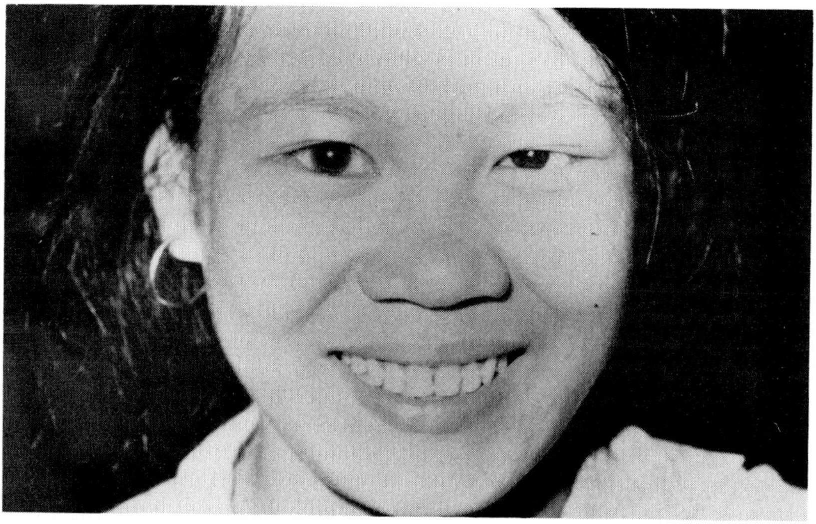

FIG. 13. South Vietnamese girl was fitted with a stock prosthesis after the insertion of a 16-mm implant.

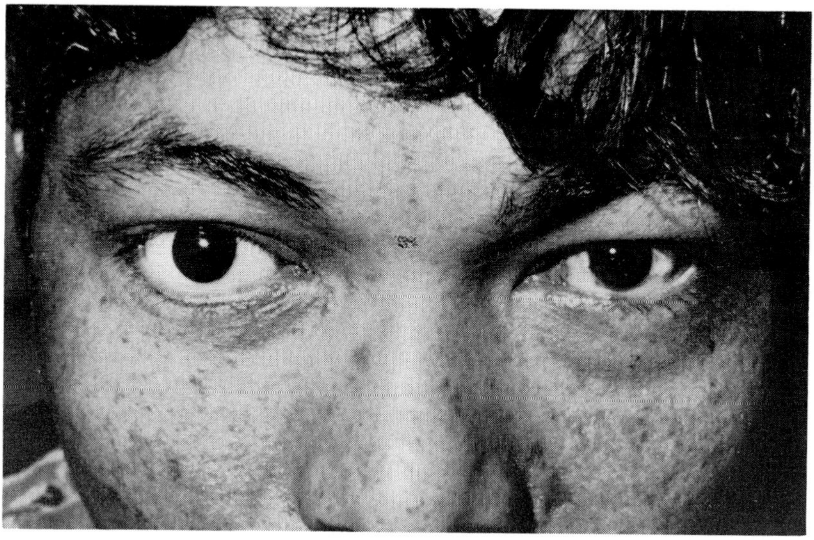

FIG. 14. Although Americans were fitted in the United States with ocular prostheses, this 18-year-old South Vietnamese soldier was fitted by a stock prosthesis sent by friends to author. A prosthesis is in place in right eye.

Summary

Severe ocular injuries accounted for 6%-9% of all war injuries in South Vietnam. All attempts were made to salvage injured eyes regardless of the visual status. Anophthalmia from the Vietnam conflict is a huge and serious problem. Thousands of American soldiers with visual impairment and blindness have returned to civilian life from Vietnam. The ophthalmologist and ocularist must be prepared to rehabilitate these men. In addition, steps should be taken to assist the South Vietnamese with their tragic problems of anophthalmia.

References

1. Tredici, T. J.: Management of opthalmic casualties in Southeast Asia: Milit. Med., vol. 133, no. 5, May 1968.
2. Vietnam Casualty Statistics, U.S. Department of Defense, 1 January 1961 to 30 December 1972.
3. Hornblass, A.: Ocular war injuries in South Vietnam. Surg. Forum, 24:500, 1973.
4. Bellow, J. G.: Observations on 300 consecutive cases of ocular war injuries. Amer. J. Ophthal., 30:309, 1947.
5. Hull, F. E.: Management of eye casualties in the Far East Command during the Korean conflict. Trans. Amer. Acad. Ophthal. Otolaryng., 56:885, 1951.
6. Hoegle, F. B.: Initial treatment of eye injuries First Corps area of Vietnam. Arch. Ophthal., 79:33, 1968.
7. McKinlay, R. T. and Cohen, D. N.: Modern concepts in ophthalmic casualty management. Ann. Ophthal., 5:1221, 1973.
8. Gombos, G. M.: Ocular war injuries in Jerusalem during the 1967 Arab-Israeli conflict Amer. J. Ophthal., 68:474, 1969.
9. Ophthalmic injuries. *In* Proceedings of CIMCPAC Fourth Conference on War Surgery, Feb. 1970.

The Mystery of the Lower Lid

Fritz Jardon

The ocularist is concerned with upper and lower lids. Although we tolerate a slight ptosis and mild increased lid fold over the prosthesis, we cannot tolerate trichiasis, an extropion or eversion and watering, nor an entropion or inversion with trichiasis and constant mucous discharge associated with lower lid deformities. The lower lid must be physiologically stable in order to maintain prosthesis position and horizontal centering.

Five basic problems creating droopy lower lids are (1) shifted implants on babies; (2) shifted implants on adults (too large/too small); (3) accidents; (4) alkali burns, adhesions or contracted orbits; and (5) badly designed, badly fitted prostheses.

The solution to the problems of the lower lid begins with a good surgical procedure to create good cul-de-sacs. The following surgical procedure for cosmetic enucleation has been outlined by Lorand V. Johnson, M.D., Professor Emeritus at Case Western Reserve University, Cleveland, Ohio:

1. Cut the recti muscles with a knife, leaving a tab of sclera to prevent retraction into the sheath.
2. Cut the nerve with the tip of the scissors not near the hinge, to prevent the cutting of a rent in posterior Tenon's capsule. Such a rent will allow immediate migration of the implant.
3. Horizontal closure of the conjunctiva is used to add tissue to the outer and inner fornix. Purse-string closure of the conjunctiva will obliterate the semilunar fold and outer canthus.
4. Too much traction on the superior rectus will depress the elevator muscle and cause a depressed upper lid fold.
5. The flat nasal edge of the conformer should be 2 mm longer than for the final fitted eye, to obtain a good lateral "overhang" to cover the lateral edge of the prosthesis.

Fritz Jardon, Ocularist, Assistant Professor, Department of Ophthalmology, Wayne State University, Detroit, Mich.

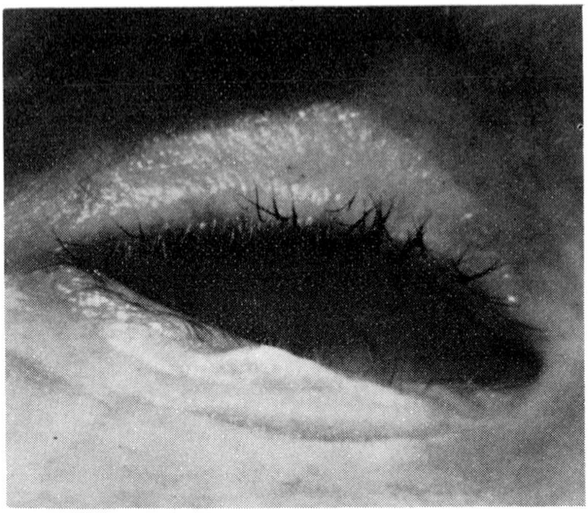

FIG. 1. Entropion and shallow cul-de-sacs.

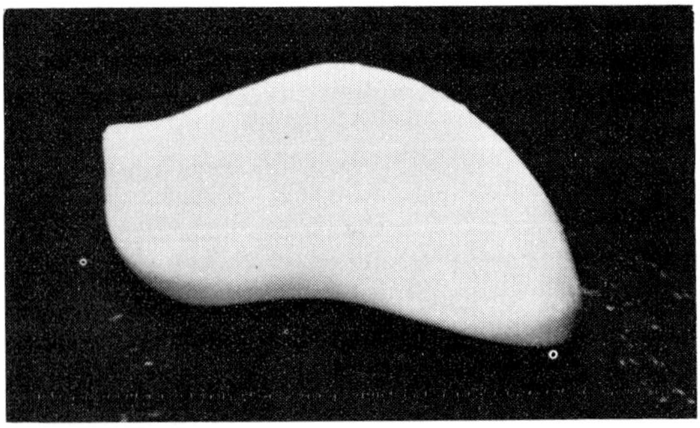

FIG. 2. Lateral view – curves of working model.

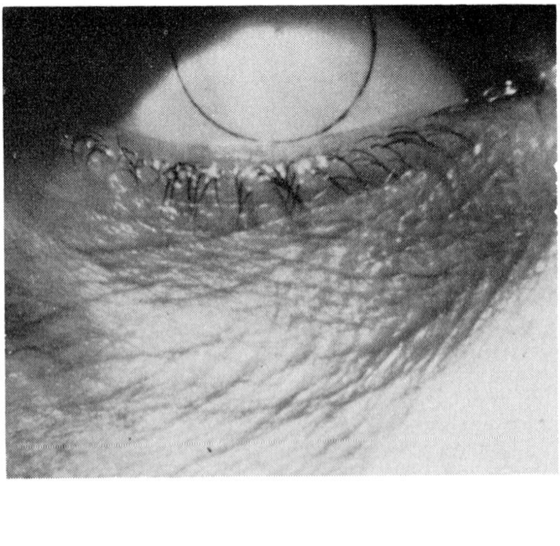

FIG. 3. Working model in socket for iris positioning.

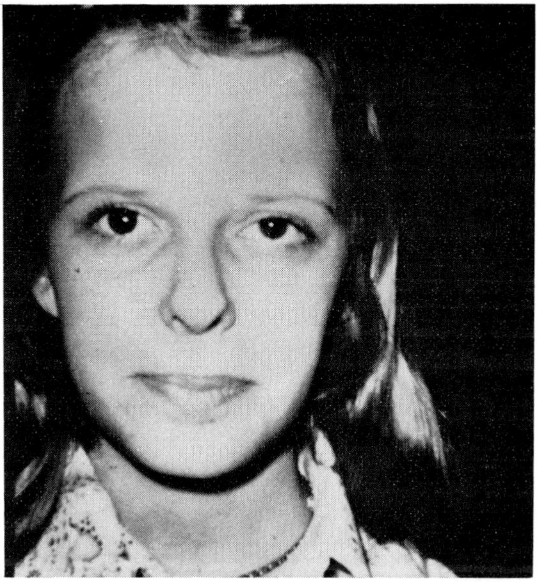

FIG. 4. Left prosthesis in place.

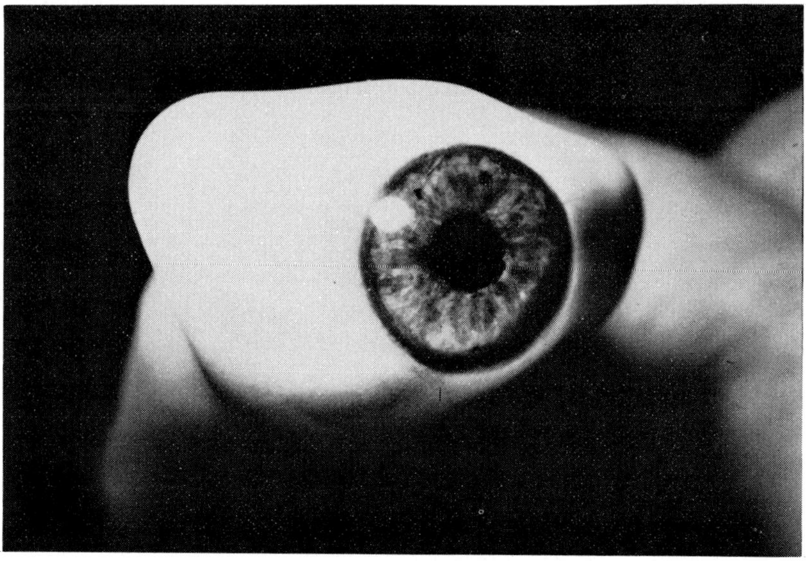

FIG. 5. Finished eye showing contour curves.

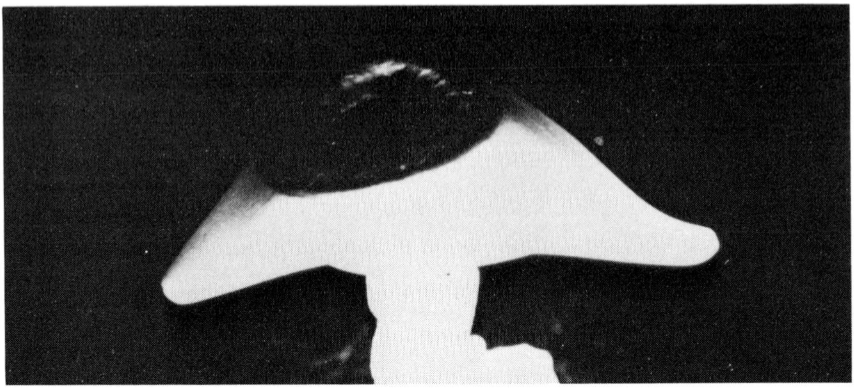

FIG. 6. Inferior and anterior eye contours.

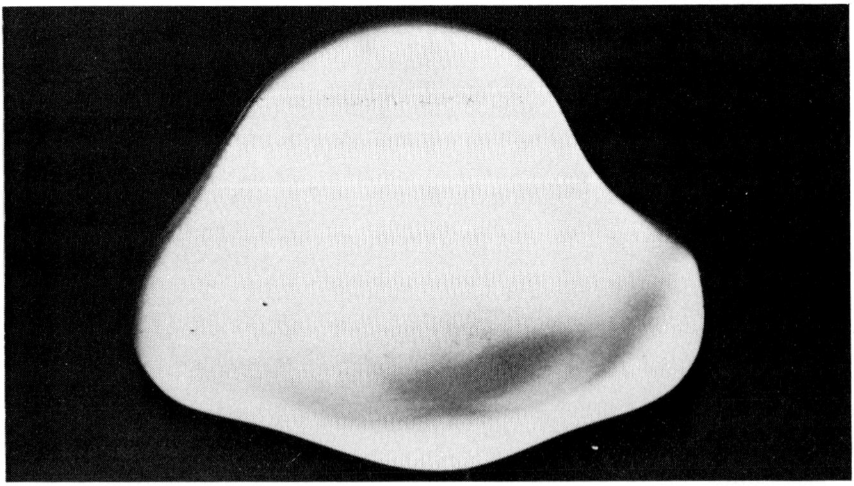

FIG. 7. Posterior view of finished eye.

6. With surgical insertion of the MOLD-A-FORM eye, the *socket is shaped* to receive an identically shaped prosthesis, to form a good upper and lower cul-de-sac and outer canthus.

Prosthesis designs and end results are shown in Figures 1-7.

A Singular View (Book Review)

O. Robert Levy

A Singular View begins with a resoundingly positive answer to a patient's most worrisome question: "Will I ever be able to lead a normal life again?"

Frank B. Brady has written a superb and truly comprehensive book detailing the problems and pitfalls facing newly monocular patients. He guides his readers through the rudimentary mechanics of a return to normalcy by the use of photographs, simple drawings, charts, lucid text and many personal anecdotes.

The physician is aware of the many adjustments that will be encountered, but the newly one-eyed patient is not. Mr. Brady enumerates some factors of utmost importance in the education of a newly monoculared patient.

Eye dominance is a factor in the adjustment period. If the dominant eye is lost, as was the case of Mr. Brady, the readjustment period will be longer and more difficult.

Visual acuity is another important factor. If there is good vision even though the remaining eye is the secondary one, less time will be required to take on the functions of the lost eye. If there is poor vision and the remaining eye is the secondary one, much more time and effort are needed in the adjustment period.

The younger the patient is the better, since youthfulness tends to indicate flexibility. Thus age is a factor which cannot be overlooked.

The length of time involved in the loss of the eye affects a patient's success. If the eye is lost through slow deterioriation, it is easier on the patient than if there is a sudden loss.

Each individual's needs or wants, his occupation and hobbies are determinants of his future success in adapting to his loss and the time necessary to do so. The psychological reactions of patients vary the total spectrum from "What's the use of living?" to "I hardly notice the difference." Mr. Brady considered his own loss as a nuisance rather than a handicap!

O. Robert Levy, Ocularist, Los Angeles, Calif.

The physician can help his patient adapt more rapidly to his loss of an eye with some counseling. (A recent survey reports that the average physician thinks he spends as much as five to eight minutes per patient appointment on counseling, but actually spends only 90 seconds per patient appointment.) Also, the physician with binocular vision, though aware of the academic, physical and emotional problems of the newly monocular-visioned person, really does not know how to teach his patient the necessary mechanics of stepping off curbs, shaking hands, pouring coffee, driving a car, etc.

Part of the educational process for the newly nonocular patient in helping to speed up his adaptation to a more comfortable environment should be to acquaint him with the actual physical changes that occur inside his head. He lists the three major things that have happened:

1. The horizontal field of vision has narrowed.
2. The depth perception has been impaired.
3. The whole visual system, including brain and motor functions, is in disarray and needs programming.

The author also gives definite examples of how the monocular person can learn to adapt more readily in sports, driving, flying, sailing and plain viewing of stationary objects. Frank Brady is not a physician. He is an engineer who learned the hard way, after losing his dominant eye when a Mallard duck crashed through the window of a research DC-3 which he was copiloting during World War II. His own remarkable adaptation was made almost without the benefit of guidance. There was none available at that time – nor was there until he decided to write this manual for the newly one-eyed.

A Singular View (published by Medical Economics Co., a division of Litton Publications) was written in careful consultation with ophthalmologits and contains a foreword by Dr. John W. McTigue, Chief of Ophthalmology at the Washington, D. C. Medical Center. Mr. Brady is director of airport equipment programs in the Research and Engineering Branch of Singer-General Precision, Inc. He has written a number of articles on electronic navigational and instrument landing aids. His first writing outside his own highly technical field is *A Singular View.* He has written this book for doctors and their patients in nontechnical language for use as a tool and a manual in avoiding the dangers and embarrassments omnipresent for the newly one-eyed person.

V. Workshop

Workshop: Complications of Enucleation

Frank O. McGehee, Jr., M.D. and George Constance

Early infection usually will lead to implant rejection. The main causes of infection are the use of a nonsterilized implant or conformer and use of improper surgical technique. The first sign of infection may be cystic formation along the conjunctival incision site. Prolapse of the conjunctiva because of chemosis may occur with an associated discharge. Late evidence of an infection is characterized by a gradual increase of socket discharge associated with a tender, inflamed conjunctival surface. The inflammation may result from either implant tilting or an improperly fitting prosthesis. Both conditions may cause pressure-point necrosis leading to a dead space and the buildup of stagnant tears.

How often should a prosthesis be cleaned? If there are no secretions or signs of an improper fit, the less handling, the better. When it is necessary to remove the prosthesis, a salt solution should be used to flush the prosthesis while it is in the socket, prior to removal. Proper hygiene by the patient should be observed.

The prosthesis itself become a source for infection. Mr. Lee Allen has noticed a foul odor when the prosthesis is incised. He has shown that acrylic implants definitely can absorb moisture in their molecular structure and thereby harbor bacteria.

Superior sulcus defects occur when the posterior orbital volume is not replaced following enucleation, leading to contracture and shrinkage of the posterior orbital tissue. Later, gravitation of the contracted muscle cone further increases the defect which is already present. These changes occur most rapidly when an orbital implant is not used. Also, there is a tendency for both enophthalmos and upper lid ptosis to occur secondarily. These same defects can occur more slowly because of atrophy of orbital fat

---

Frank O. McGehee, Jr., M.D., Ophthalmologist; and George Constance, Ocularist, Houston, Texas.

resulting from migration of the implant itself. Preventive measures include using a large enough implant and positioning it as far posteriorly as possible, as Dr. Robert Soll has described. Increased traction against gravity can be obtained by suturing the superior rectus muscle into the upper fornix. Support from below the implant can be achieved by suturing the inferior oblique muscle to the lateral rectus muscle.

What type of implant is best for correction of a superior sulcus defect? For small defects, subperiosteal implantation of glass beads can be used. For those cases associated with enophthalmos, Dr. Soll's expandable subperiosteal implant is an excellent choice. Solid silicone implants, even when wired to the inferior orbital rim, have a tendency to extrude. Mr. Allen has suggested the use of a prosthetic shelf which can be custom made to correct a superior sulcus defect. This also corrects the pseudoptosis. However, correction of a true ptosis by modification of a prosthesis is difficult.

True ptosis may occur by itself or with a superior sulcus defect. By using the Allen technique, pseudoptosis can be ruled out. The correction of true ptosis is primarily surgical, consisting of a levator aponeurosis plication as suggested by Dr. Richard Tenzil. A full-thickness block of lid skin also can be excised, depending upon the patient's cosmetic appearance. The upper lid may retract following the implantation surgical procedure if the levator muscle is sutured by mistake. A scleral graft extension from the levator aponeurosis to the tarsus is the proper surgical approach for correction of a superior lid recession.

An implant extrusion may occur immediately following enucleation or sometime later. Pressure on the incision site can occur from either an oversized implant or too large a conformer. If no secondary infection is present, then immediate replacement is desirable, using a smaller implant. Repeated extrusion may occur if the implant is too large. If needed, donor or preserved sclera can be used to cover a defect in Tenon's capsule.

If the tissues are traumatized, socket contraction may occur after implant extrusion. Therefore, attention should be given to the condition of the socket before replacement of the implant. If socket reconstruction is done, several months should elapse to allow complete healing to take place before reinserting another orbital implant.

In another surgical approach, described by Dr. Charles Iliff, an implant is replaced through a brow incision. In this procedure, a hollow silicone implant is first inserted and then inflated to the proper size with either antibiotic or saline solution.

Contraction of the fornices may occur due to absence of the conformer or downward migration of the implant, which causes tissue adherence of the socket lining to the floor of the orbit. In either case, surgical expansion of the fornices is necessary before a prosthesis can be properly fitted. Contraction of the fornices can cause the lower lid to turn inward, preventing the prosthesis from staying in position. The inferior fornix then must be expanded with a mucous membrane graft before a prosthesis can be fitted properly.

An entropion of the lower lid must not be confused with that of a recessed lower lid. The latter condition would require scleral grafting instead of an entropion procedure. Occasionally a tendency toward an ectropion may occur because of the weight of the prosthesis and laxity of the lower lid.

Orbital asymmetry is a late complication when enucleation is done in the preadolescent patient. At this age level, even when both an implant and conformer are used, the orbital bone growth is slowed. In an effort to minimize the asymmetry, graduated sizes of conformers should be used until no further expansion of the socket is possible. Following adolescence, the socket may be enlarged, if necessary, by mucous membrane grafting. It has been suggested that squeezing exercises with a conformer in place may help to expand the preadolescent socket. In reality, this only causes hypertrophy of the orbicularis muscle, which could lead to an ectropion instead.

In summary, seven major complications have been discussed in an effort to improve the results of enucleation surgical procedures.

VI. Scientific Exhibits

Scientific Exhibits

A CONTEMPORARY IRIS REPRODUCTION TECHNIQUE. *Charles L. Workman*, Ocularist, Milwaukee, Wisc.

This colorful exhibit described a contemporary method most commonly used by ocularists to paint artificial irides for ocular prostheses. Eight panels took the viewer through the steps necessary to reproduce a human iris from the raw ingredients to the finished result.

The first panel was a collage of the actual materials used. A small palette ablaze with nine artists' oil colors was at the upper left of the panel. (Several ocularists use dry pigments instead of oils.) Next to the palette were two bottles; one contained methyl-methacrylate monomer and the other a mixture of three parts monomer to one part methyl-methacrylate polymer resin, which forms a syrup. The syrup is a base to which the oil pigments are added, providing a fast-drying medium. It can be lightly tinted for translucency or more heavily tinted to make it opaque. Therefore, the medium lends an aura of dimension to a flat surface. Toward the lower section of the collage were two sizes of small red sable brushes and a mixing dish; a black vinyl disk on which the color mixture is painted; and a clear acrylic cornea-pupil piece with stem. The disk and cornea-pupil piece are cemented together when color matching of the human iris is completed.

For demonstration purposes, six black plastic disks, 4 inches in diameter, were placed on the second through seventh panels to describe how the color is applied to the disk in approximately six layers. The observer could see how each step would gradually transform the black disk into the pattern and hues of a hazel-blue human iris. Because the pigments can be regulated within the medium as to the extent of translucency, the first layers show through as vividly as the last.

The exhibitor pointed out that contrast is also important in creating the illusion of depth and dimension when forming the striation pattern. The black disk provided the basic ingredient for this illusion, demonstrated in the first step by the use of titanium-white paint layered over the surface. The evolution continued in subsequent steps as general color tones of blue and yellow ochre were added. Components such as collarette and limbal ring were sketched lightly in white to establish their relationship to pupil and iris size. Then the final hues of the limbus and collarette were added, first in softer browns or greys and later in stronger, richer tones where emphasis was needed. As the steps came closer to the point of completion, the exhibitor mentioned the importance of darkening the hues nearest the pupil and softening those near the limbus. This was done to overcome distortions and magnification caused by cementing the cornea-pupil piece onto the colored disk.

The last panel was a large photograph of the patient whose iris had been reproduced. It was strategically placed next to the seventh panel showing the excellently matched final reproduction in enlarged detail and actual size.

HYGENIC CARE OF THE PROSTHESIS. *Joseph W. Soper* and *George Constance*, Ocularists, Houston, Texas.

Hygenic care of the prosthesis, although not difficult for the patient to follow, is vitally important to the patient's comfort, appearance and success in wearing the ocular prosthesis. The ocularist should advise the patient of the factors involved in maintaining good hygenic habits, although his recommendations should only be given with the complete agreement of the referring ophthalmologist – which should be a predetermined, ongoing arrangement.

On a routine basis, the patient should return to the ocularist every six months for prosthetic evaluation. On this visit a complete evaluation should be made by the ocularist of the prosthesis and the general condition of the socket. The following factors should be considered when examining the prosthesis.

To ensure that a proper finished surface is maintained, the ocularist should check for scratches on the anterior and posterior surfaces. If any scratches or rough areas are found, pumicing of the surfaces should be done, followed by reglazing. The cause of the scratches should be investigated and the patient instructed in future care so the scratches do not reoccur. A notation should be made on the patient's record concerning the location, type of scratches and the instructions given to the patient. At the completion of the resurfacing and glazing, the prosthesis should have its original glaze and life-like appearance. During the visit, the fit of the prosthesis and overall cosmetic appearance are evaluated and noted in the record. Indicated modifications in the fit are made or intention of possible future modifications is noted.

Socket secretions in correct amounts are desirable, although they may be excessive or insufficient. This most important factor of prosthetic comfort is evaluated on each visit. If the socket is red and irritated, secretions will most likely be excessive. Factors which can cause excessive secretions include (1) poor fit, (2) poor surface and edge finish, (3) poor glaze, (4) patient handling and contamination of the prosthesis, (5) irritation from frequent insertion and removal, (6) excessive prosthetic size restricting lid closure, (7) excessive vault over the socket causing a pocket to trap secretions, and (8) chemical irritation of the socket.

Dry sockets can be aided by using lubricants such as Enucleene, Tearisol, Ocular Tear, odorless castor oil (an excellent lubricant) and

Liquifilm Tears. Frequently, though, these lubricants are used in excessive secretion cases when they are not necessary. In many of these cases the surface and glaze of the prosthesis need correcting.

It should be stressed that the prosthesis should not be removed by the patient, as a well-fitted and glazed prosthesis can be worn for months without removal. The six-month follow-up visit is a must and is most important to the patient for total comfort and hygiene of the prosthesis. This check-up not only will provide the patient proper hygenic care but also will keep both the patient and ocularist aware of any problems and changes that may develop.

PATHOLOGICAL AND ATYPICAL CONDITIONS IN THE PROSTHETIC EYE. *Phillip A. Danz*, Ocularist, San Francisco, Calif.

This exhibit presented some two hundred glass-bulb-replica prosthetic eyes simulating various eye diseases. These excellently fabricated eyes were extremely life-like and accurate in their duplication of the coloring and anatomy of the diseases.

The pathological eye kit was created in the 1880s by Amandus Mueller in Germany. The kit has been handed down through four generations of the Danz-Mueller family to Phillip and Ted Danz of San Francisco. Only four of these kits were manufactured, so it is priceless. The prosthetic pathological eye specimens were fabricated in order to instruct medical doctors of that period. The specimens were blown from observation of actual pathological conditions.

This pathological eye kit was presented to demonstrate the consummate skill of the glass blowing of that period and to offer the idea of using pathological eye kits as a teaching aid for medical and paramedical personnel.

In addition, a much smaller pathological eye kit was presented which consisted of acrylic prosthetic eyes simulating the following atypical conditions that the ocularist may see in his practice: (1) cataract, (2) coloboma of the iris, (3) arcus senilis, (4) mydriasis, (5) keratoconus, (6) corneal scarring, (7) dermoid tumor, and (8) conjunctivitis.

The glass pathological eye kit currently resides at the University of California Medical Center, Division of Ophthalmology, San Francisco.

PTOSIS AND THE TARSUS.* *Lee Allen, Ocularist*, The University of Iowa Hospitals and Clinics, Iowa City.

The exhibit consisted of a 5X lifesize silicone rubber model of the tarsus and palpebral ligaments of the upper eyelid, suspended on a panel in such a manner that each viewer could manipulate the model in a number of ways while observing the changes in position of the upper edge of the "tarsus" and the position and contour of the "lid margin." Directions to the sides of the model tarsus requested the visitor to "Elevate me," "Depress me," "Tilt me" and "Twist me."

The text of the exhibit called attention to the similarity of the tarsus and ligaments to an inverted hammock. Similarity was drawn between the points of insertion of the palpebral ligaments and the hooks or points of support of a hammock. The leather-like character of the tarsus was mentioned and related to the way in which the entire tarsus rotates around the axis through its points of support.

This exhibit was conceived and designed specifically to compliment the paper, "Reduction of Upper Eyelid Ptosis with the Prosthesis, with Special Attention to a Recently Devised, More Effective Method," given by Lee Allen before the scientific session of the society. That paper is included in this present volume.

The importance of the tarsus in correction of ptosis by complex mechanical principles in design of the prosthesis, rather than by the ineffective method of fitting larger prostheses, will be best understood from careful reading of the paper. The most important single point to be gained from both the paper and the exhibit is that space must be maintained or created at the posterior aspect of the upper surface of the prosthesis into which the upper edge of the tarsus may rotate when the eyelid margin is elevated.

As supplementary observations, twisting and tilting of the model tarsus revealed how the projected contour of the eyelid margin may be made to elevate on one side and drop on the other in order to achieve the desired balance with the companion eye.

---

*Given the Best Scientific Exhibit Award for 1974.

SCLERAL COSMETIC SHELLS AND LENSES. *Joseph W. Michel*, Ocularist, Philadelphia, Pa.

Most ground work for the contemporary cosmetic prosthesis was accomplished by contact lens pioneers. Techniques were refined for fitting scleral lenses to sighted eyes which resulted in the development of the flush-fitting therapeutic scleral lenses for traumatic and pathological anterior segment problems.

The prosthesis may be totally opaque and be referred to as a scleral cosmetic shell, or it may contain optics and be referred to as a scleral cosmetic lens. In either case, the fitting of a patient with a scleral shell or lens can be very gratifying to both the patient and the ocularist.

This intriguing educational exhibit of 16 beautiful full-color, framed photographs was uniquely displayed on two revolving turntables. Accompanying the display was an interesting treatise which followed the history of the scleral cosmetic prosthesis and included the methods by which the scleral cosmetic prosthesis should be used for the maximum benefit of the patient, such as the fact that acceptable candidates should first be fitted with a clear plastic lens of optimum fit. The term "optimum fit" goes beyond the areas of thickness and size considered for a basic scleral lens – if the finished lens is to be transparent, it does not matter if there is space between the edge of the lens and the inner canthus; but if the lens is to be colored for cosmetic purposes, this space becomes conspicuous and undesirable. Therefore, it is important to make the clear lens as long as possible nasally without discomfort or dislocation on excursions. It was pointed out that selection of patients should be done by the ophthalmologist.

The lens can be either the minimum-clearance, fluidless type (fenestrated with corneal clearance) or the flush-fitting type. If the cornea is not anesthetic, the minimum type is indicated. If there is little or no corneal sensitivity, then the flush-fitting lens is the proper choice.

When the clear scleral lens has optimum fit and the patient can tolerate it for a full day of wearing, it can then be colored to match cosmetically the patient's fellow eye.

Since there is such a wide variety of eyes which run the gamut from microphthalmic to exophthalmic and from blind to photophobic, the treatise also included the following outline of indications in order to offer some help in determining the type of scleral lens/shell required:

Traumatic injury to globe requires:
- Scleral cosmetic lens, with or without optics, as indicated.

Globe micropthalmia requires:
- Minimum-clearance scleral lens thick enough to equalize palpebral fissures; cosmetic conversion if appearance is abnormal; optics when there is residual sight.

Diplopia requires:
- Opaque corneal lens to occlude one eye or scleral lens with pupil partially occluded, for monocular diplopia.

Scleral evisceration requires:
- Scleral cosmetic lens, flush fitting.

Albinism requires:
- Pair of corneal cosmetic lenses; scleral cosmetics if more opacity needed, with small pupil aperture.

Polycoria requires:
- Corneal cosmetic lens if lens centers over desired pupil; scleral cosmetic lens if preferred pupil is not in corneal center.

Extraocular muscle amblyopia requires:
- Opaque corneal cosmetic lens to occlude better eye.

Aberration of crystalline lens distorting vision requires:
- Complete occliesion with opaque corneal cosmetic or occlusion of distracting image with scleral lens and partial pupil.

This outline was aptly illustrated with close-up "before and after" color photographs.

SURGICAL CORRECTION OF ANOPHTHALMIC ENOPHTHALMOS.

William L. Walter, M.D., St. Louis Eye Clinic, St. Louis, Mo.

This exhibit was a twelve minute audio-visual presentation of the surgical technique used by the author to correct the orbital deformities (ie, deepened supratarsal suclus, pseudoptosis of upper eyelid and enophthalmos of prosthesis) which can develop following the removal of a patient's eye. The operation consists of the subperiosteal implantation of multiple small, round, 5-mm glass beads near the apex of the orbit by a lateral canthal approach. Certain phases of the bead implant operation, which was described by Smith, Obear and Leone in 1967, have been changed slightly by the author, and these modifications were presented.

One modification was the use of a specially made instrument for inserting metal beads which was helpful in accurately placing the glass beads near the orbital apex. Another change of the surgical technique, re-attaching the lateral canthal tendon at a higher level, was described in order to correct the associated orbital deformities of later canthus displacement and sagging of the lower eyelid margin which can also be present in cases of anophthalmic enophthalmos.

Preoperative and postoperative views of seven patients who had their orbital deformities corrected by the subperiosteal insertion of glass beads were presented. The cosmetic results in each case were very good, and no complications were encountered. The exhibit demonstrated that the accurate placement of glass beads at the orbital apex can be very helpful in treating patients with anophthalmic enophthalmos and associated orbital deformities. The surgical results were quite gratifying, making this particular surgical technique an important one to be included in the armamentarium of the oculoplastic surgeon for treating these orbital deformities.

Subject Index